Pasture Perfect

The Far-Reaching Benefits of Choosing Meat, Eggs, and Dairy Products from Grass-Fed Animals

By Jo Robinson

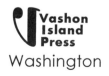

Vashon
Island
Press

Washington

PASTURE PERFECT
By Jo Robinson

Text and illustrations copyright © 2004 by Jo Robinson

First paperback printing, 2004

Robinson, Jo, 1947–

Pasture Perfect:
The Far-Reaching Benefits of Choosing Meat, Eggs, and Dairy Products from Grass-Fed Animals

Includes bibliographical references and index.
ISBN 0-9678116-1-9

160 pages

Printed in the United States of America by Vashon Island Press

Vashon Island Press
29428 129th Ave S.W.
Vashon WA 98070
1-866-453-8489

Cover photo taken by David Schafer,
Schafer Farms Natural Meats, Missouri.

Book and cover design by Frances Robinson

Printed on recycled paper

A Note to the Reader:

One of the challenges in writing a science-based book for the public is knowing how extensively to document the manuscript. Some readers want a reference for every major point. Others want the meat of the story, not the scientific underpinnings. I've tried to work out a compromise. I have provided references for the most important or controversial statements, but not all the studies. If you want more references, I refer you to a comprehensive bibliography on my website, *www.eatwild.com*. Look for the "Scientific References" section.

My previous book, *Why Grassfed Best!* listed contact information for 50 pasture-based producers. I was unable to list suppliers in this book because there are now over 500 of them. Go to *www.eatwild.com* for an up-to-date directory that is organized by state. You can also visit the website for more detailed information about all the topics in this book and for news updates as well.

Go Grass!

"Land, then, is not merely soil; it is a fountain of energy flowing through a circuit of soils, plants, and animals."

—Aldo Leopold, 1949

"Society is closing a circle and returning to a radical concept: nature has the best ideas. In the long run, nature's models are the only ones that are truly sustainable ecologically and economically. Raising grazing animals on grass, especially if they are herded in a natural manner, is a model that works unquestionably for the health of the land, its people, and its animals."

—Courtney White, Executive Director,
The Quivira Coalition

"In the beginning, we ranched like everyone else, which means we lost money. We changed directions in the 1990s and began finishing our steers on pasture. Now, we're making a profit selling our grass-fed meat to neighbors, local stores, and restaurants. When local people are supporting local agriculture, you know you're doing something right."

—David and Kay James, The James Ranch,
Durango, Colorado

"The 'good' fatty acids, collectively known as Omega-3 and conjugated linoleic (CLA), are in short supply in the modern American diet, and one may be well advised to take advantage of sources which provide them, such as the meat and dairy products of grass-fed animals."

—Bill Elkins, M.D., Associate Professor Emeritus,
Department of Pathology,
University of Pennsylvania School of Medicine

"Overuse of antibiotics in animal agriculture continues to erode the effectiveness of antibiotics used in human medicine. Moving animals out of confinement and onto pastures results in far less use of antibiotics. The more animals we grow on pasture, the better it is for public health."

—Margaret Mellon, M.D., Union of Concerned Scientists

"While I don't subscribe to panaceas, grass-based animal production is pretty damn close; if we are serious about creating farming systems that protect the environment, human health, animal well-being, local communities, AND farmer profitability, then we must get serious about promoting pasture production in every region of this country. If we want to get serious about stemming the tides of family farm loss, childhood obesity, hypoxia in the Gulf, biotech in our food, and factory hog production, grass is the ticket. Begin to visualize the Midwest planted back to grass and all you see is health! GO Grass!!"

—Tim Bowser, Executive Director, FoodRoutes Network

"Consumers and chefs across the country are intrigued by the benefits of pasture-based agriculture. Animals that are raised on grass have a fresh and natural diet and a low-stress environment. As a result, the animals are healthier and provide higher quality products. A production system that is good for the animals, the environment, and consumers is a win-win-win proposition. Just as important, it provides a profitable business for independent farmers."

—Jim Ennis, Program Director, Midwest Food Alliance

"We have to go back to Mother Nature's way of doing things, and until we do that we're going to continue to go down in every way possible. In farming, if it's not sustainable, we shouldn't be doing it."

—Willie Nelson

"Grass-based farming is the one bright spot in agriculture today."

—Terry Gompert, Extension Educator, University of Nebraska

"I farmed the wrong way for 40 years. I was at the mercy of the chemical and seed industries and the misguided people at the university. I worked 17 hours a day and couldn't support my family. At the point that I sold my dairy cows, I was earning 42 cents an hour. Now I'm straightened out. I'm raising cows on pasture."

—Connecticut Dairy Farmer

"Grass-based farming is financially viable for farmers, great for the land, and friendly to nearby rural businesses. Odors are minimized, the landscape is esthetically pleasing, and the products are a healthy addition to our diets. Buy your animal products from stewards who raise their animals on high-quality pasture. And while you are at it, enjoy what you are eating. You are contributing to health in more ways than you know."

—George Boody, Executive Director,
Land Stewardship Project

"Growing animals on pasture has the potential to preserve the biodiversity of our agricultural lands, as well as reduce other environmental impacts such as global climate change and air and water pollution from agriculture."

—Dr. Rita Schenck, Executive Director, Institute for Environmental Research and Education

"Dr. Martin Luther King, Jr. said 'And there comes a time when one must take a position that is neither safe, nor politic, nor popular—but one must take it simply because it is right.' Good conscience would dictate that raising animals on pasture is the logical choice in achieving a globally sustainable food system."

—Rick Hopkins, President, American Pasturage, Inc.

"We have succeeded in industrializing the beef calf, transforming what was once a solar-powered ruminant into the very last thing we need: another fossil-fuel machine."

—Michael Pollan, "Power Steer," *The New York Times*

"All flesh is grass, and the goodliness thereof is as the flower of the field."

—Isaiah 40

Contents

Preface

As this book goes to press, I am pleased and surprised by the number of people who are now buying their meat, eggs, and dairy products from farmers who raise their animals on pasture. Tens of thousands of shoppers are willing to spend more time and effort getting their food and pay a little more in the bargain. Once they've tried products from grass-fed animals, they're reluctant to go back. They've discovered food that enhances their health, delights their taste buds, and gives them a deeper sense of connection to the natural world.

Four years ago, when I wrote *Why Grassfed Is Best!*, the prototype of this book, few people knew about the benefits of products from grass-fed animals. In fact, to many people, the term "grass-fed" had a negative connotation. The assumption was that the meat would be dry, tough, or "gamey." The term "grain-fed," on the other hand, was viewed as a mark of quality. If you wanted tender and juicy meat, you bought meat from animals raised in the feedlots and fattened on corn. At the time, there were also very few suppliers of pastured products. In 2000, I could locate only 50 farmers who were selling their grass-fed products directly to consumers and most of them got the bulk of their income from other sources.

Today, grassfarming is the talk of the town. There may be more than 1,000 grass-based producers in the United States and Canada, and still the demand exceeds the supply. The media has been helping to fan the fires. In the last two years, pasture-based farming has been featured in *The Smithsonian, The New York Times, The Wall Street Journal, The Atlantic Monthly, The San Francisco Chronicle, The Dallas Morning News, The Los Angeles Times, House and Garden, Wine Spectator, Mother Earth News,* and *The National Review.*

Why this sudden interest in grass-fed products? Although the demand seems to have sprung up overnight, people have been laying down the groundwork for decades. Environmentalists have been recommending putting animals out to pasture as a way to reduce pollution, cut down on the use of fossil fuel, and prevent the erosion of top soil. People who work with farmers have been encouraging them to feed more grass and less grain to their animals as a way to lower the cost of production. And animal welfare advocates have viewed pasture-based farming as a way to improve conditions for the animals.

But these three benefits were not enough to create a market for grass-fed products. Something was missing. What few people knew at the time is that products from animals raised on pasture are better for our health than conventional products. This is a benefit that would speak directly to consumers.

I helped dredge up some of the nutritional information. As a freelance writer, I had narrowed my focus to health and nutrition. I was especially interested in the differences between our original diet—wild plants, seafood, and game—and our modern diet. Research was showing that the more primitive diet is better for our health in almost all ways.

Clearly, it wasn't possible for hundreds of millions of us to head back to the woods and live as hunter gatherers. But it might be possible to eat food that resembled the hunter-gatherer diet. I first got a glimmer of this when I found a study showing that meat from cattle raised on grass was very similar to wild game. My interest was piqued. What else was known about food from grass-fed animals?

Not much, I soon discovered. Most of our modern research studies grain-fed animals raised in confinement, the status quo. To find information about grass-based production, I had to unearth studies published before the advent of factory farming; read journals from the few countries that still raise their animals on pasture; and read every relevant U.S. study I could find. In some instances, I even had to rely on laboratory tests funded by the farmers themselves.

Eventually, I rounded up about a hundred studies showing that products from grass-fed animals are better for human health. When this information was added to the fact that grass-based farming is better for the animals, the environment, and family farmers, it was a win-win-win-win proposition.

The first time I shared my information with a large group of people was in November, 1999, when I gave a talk to 500 ranchers at a grazing conference organized by grass guru Allan Nation. Most of the attendees were "cow-calf operators." Being a cow-calf operator means that you raise a herd of cows on pasture, breed them, and then let the calves run with their mothers until the calves are old enough to be shipped to the feedlots. This is the sunny side of the beef industry. But the moment the calves are loaded into trucks and transported off your ranch, they are swept up into the feedlot system. Welcome to the dark side.

I remember feeling a flush of anxiety as I stood at the podium arranging my overheads. I had never talked to such a large group of people before, never to so many men, and never to a room full of ranchers with their 18-inch biceps crossed over their chests. Odds were good that I was about to say something that would expose my near total ignorance of ranching. I had learned a lot about the benefits of grass-fed products, but very little about raising the animals themselves.

Ten minutes into my talk, I could see that I was being given the benefit of the doubt. Arms were uncrossing. People were starting to take notes. When I finished my talk and asked for questions, dozens of arms shot up in the air. One of the first questions came from a young rancher who wanted to know where he could learn more about the health benefits of grass-fed meat. In preparation for the conference, I had put together a little book titled *Why Grassfed Is Best!* that summarized my findings. I raised a copy in the air and said there were 50 more for sale just outside the ballroom.

I'll never forget what happened next. Within seconds, people were standing up and moving toward the back doors. First, only a handful of people were making an exodus. Then there were fifty and a hundred. I was confused. Was everyone rushing to buy my book or did they want to be first in line at the dinner banquet? I continued to answer questions, even though half my audience had fled.

Later, I learned what had been going on outside the doors. The people had indeed left the room to buy a copy of my book. The first ranchers to approach the sales table had stood in line. But as the line lengthened, it became obvious that there were too few books to go around. People began grabbing books, throwing their money down on the table, and making their own change. All the books were gone before the bulk of the would-be buyers had left the ballroom. Believe me, this is not a common occurrence for a freelance writer. I'm accustomed to sitting at a table at a book signing hoping that someone will come talk to me. This little book had caused a stampede.

Gradually, as I've learned more about ranching, I have begun to understand the reason for the pandemonium. Raising animals for the feedlot industry, which is the job of most ranchers today, is a precarious business. Although you may do an excellent job raising your calves, sheep, or hogs, your ability to make a profit is influenced by a host of other factors, including the weather, the global economy, outbreaks of foodborne disease, the price of feed, the cost of drugs, government subsidies, the natural ups and downs of the market cycle, the price of oil, and fluctuations in consumer demand. One year, the stars line up, and you make a decent living. The next two years, the constellations shift, and you break even or lose money. In recent decades, there have been more down years than up.

My talk about the benefits of raising animals on pasture gave some of the ranchers a vision of a more hopeful, profitable future. To them, the most important piece of information had been that raising animals on grass created healthier products for consumers. Many of them knew already that a well-run, grass-based operation could benefit the environment. And they knew from direct experience that pasture-raised animals were healthy and lived low-stress lives. But when you added the fact that the meat was more nutritious and that it was free from hormones, antibiotics, and other additives, you had a product you could take to market.

After that maiden talk, I was invited to speak to more groups of ranchers, and to people interested in animal welfare, the environment, sustainable agriculture, and the plight of family farmers. To a growing number of people, raising animals on pasture seemed like the solution to some of our most intractable agricultural problems.

Within a year, the number of grass-based producers doubled. Farmers began selling their meat, eggs, and dairy products at their farm stores and at nearby farmers' markets. Customers were driving to the farm, picking up a dozen eggs, a pound of cheese or a couple of steaks, and going home to try them out. They liked what they ate and came back for more, this time bringing a friend. The farmers bought more chicks, calves, and lambs and still sold all they could raise. More farmers went into the grassfarming business, and more people came to shop.

Today, the interest in grass-fed products has grown so steadily that it will be a number of years before the supply meets the demand. Raising animals on pasture is a go-slow operation. Before you can expand your herd, for example, you might have to lease or purchase more land and then improve the pasture. Or you might have to change your breeding program so that your animals fatten more easily on grass or produce more tender meat. Then, because you are not using growth-promoting hormones, antibiotics, or high-octane feed, you have to wait for the grass-fed animals to mature at their natural pace, which takes much longer than the factory models. As is true for excellent wine, you cannot market grass-fed products before their time—no matter how many people are clamoring for them.

The quality of the meat is improving as well. When I first began touring grass-based farms, I wasn't sure if the meat at the dinner table was going to be tender and juicy, or dry and tough. There is an art and science to producing excellent quality grass-fed meat, and not everyone had mastered it. Today, just a couple of years later, I find that most of the meat ranges from good to very good. And yes, I've eaten steaks from a handful of ranches that are superior to any grain-fed meat on the market.

A number of food critics share my assessment. In May, 2002, Marian Burros wrote in *The New York Times*, "Today, there is some grass-fed meat that is superior to the meat harvested from grain-fed animals..." Corby Krummer, writing in *The Atlantic Monthly* in the May, 2003 issue, went one step farther: "Grass-fed beef tastes better than corn-fed beef; meatier, purer, far less fatty, the way we imagine beef tasted before feedlots and farm subsidies changed ranchers and cattle." Sam Gugino, *Wine Spectator* 's Tastes columnist, reported in the August 2003 issue that a strip steak supplied by a grass-based producer was "delicious, rich and full-flavored, but without the excessive fattiness on the finish of some prime beef. The filet mignon was perhaps even more impressive, given the fact that this cut is generally chosen for tenderness, not flavor."

As pasture-based ranching grows in popularity, it's getting ever easier to buy the products. Several years ago, your only option was to drive out to a ranch and buy a quarter or half an animal. Many people still buy in bulk, but now you can also purchase individual, USDA-inspected cuts of meat on the farm, through the Internet, at farmers' markets and in specialty food stores. In a few areas of the country, such as the Big Island of Hawaii, you can walk into your local supermarket and purchase fresh, USDA-inspected, 100 percent grass-fed meat for only slightly more than you'd pay for feedlot meat.

Inevitably, the continued success of this greenest of industries will generate a new set of problems. It may be convenient to buy a grass-fed steak at your supermarket, but it severs your contact with the farmer. How are you going to know what the animals were fed and how they were treated without visiting the ranch? Lacking this direct contact, it will be necessary for the pasture-based farmers to define terms, agree on national standards, and find some way to monitor production—a time-consuming and political process.

As the market matures, there will also be increasing competition from larger enterprises. How will small-scale producers survive when Wal-Mart offers range-fed meat imported from Uruguay at half the going rate? As prices are forced down, will farmers go out of business or try to survive by cutting corners and lowering their standards?

As vexing as these problems may be, they are the right ones to be having. It's far better to be wrangling over grazing standards, definitions of terms, certification, and market share than to allow the current feedlot system to continue unchecked. As food and political activist Kenny Ausubel said at a recent conference, "If we don't change directions, we will end up precisely where we are heading." At the present time, we are hurtling toward a world where family farms are quaint relics from the past, farm workers are poorly paid and exposed to hazardous working conditions, our animals are genetically altered to satisfy corporate needs, and our meat, eggs, and dairy products contain ever more unwanted "additives" and fewer desirable nutrients.

The good news is that we are witnessing the birth of a lively countermovement. The number of pasture-based farms is on the rise. The quality of the food is improving. And the products are becoming more convenient and readily available. As tens of thousands of people treat themselves to this wholesome, nutritious, and delicious food, they are helping to save the farmers, the animals, the environment, and their own health one meal at a time. As others have said, they are doing good by eating well.

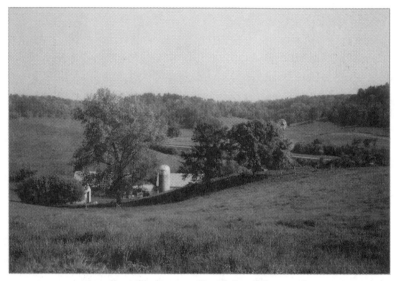

Nordic Hills Farm, Ontario, Wisconsin

Chapter 1

Imagine

I magine that you are about to tour a pasture-based farm—a farm where cattle are being raised from birth to market on high-quality grass. Unlike animals raised in a feedlot, the cattle have never been confined in close quarters, fed grain, implanted with hormones, treated routinely with antibiotics, or fed any questionable feed ingredients. They live a life very similar to life on the prairie, except that they are protected from predators and always have fresh water and high-quality food.

As you step out of your car, you notice that the air smells like grass and clover, not manure. Looking out at the green fields, you see the cattle, heads down, slowly mowing their way across the pasture. The ranch is a welcome addition to the landscape. The owners, "George and Eleanor Drake," a couple in their early forties, greet you at the car and lead you out to the pasture so you can observe the animals and learn how they manage the ranch. You follow them as they open a gate and usher you into the pasture.

The first stop on the tour brings you to a moveable rubber tank filled with fresh water. Instead of letting the cattle drink at will from their stream, potentially eroding the banks and polluting the water, the Drakes bring fresh water to the animals. Next they draw your attention to the dense thicket of bushes and trees that encircles the pasture. Unlike some ranchers, they don't use every scrap of land for farming. Their goal is to maintain a continuous ring of habitat for the local wildlife. During the eight years that they have owned the 120-acre ranch, they have documented an increase in the number of pheasants, rabbits, quail, hawks, woodpeckers, and song birds. Eleanor opens a notebook and shows you her dense record of bird sightings.

Now you are within about 200 yards of the grazing cattle. For the first time, you see a pair of llamas intermingled with the cows.

Llamas? The Drakes explain that the llamas are a part of their "predator-friendly" policy. Instead of trying to kill off the predators, they focus their efforts on protecting the herd. Their solution is to station a pair of "guard llamas" with the cattle. Llamas are known for their fiercely protective nature. When they perceive a threat, they will spit, kick, scream, and give chase. The invaders flee, leaving the calves or lambs unmolested. Other like-minded ranchers protect their animals with specially trained dogs. Some go one step farther and accept some predation as a consequence of living on the land, a voluntary wilderness tax.

Now, your attention is drawn to the grass. Eleanor and George get down on their hands and knees and point out the clover, alfalfa, and wild plants that are mixed in with the grass. Their primary job, they explain, is to provide lush pasture. The animals do the rest of the work for them. Because the grass is so vital to their operation, they refer to themselves as "grassfarmers," rather than ranchers. You learn that a critical factor in managing the grass is to regulate its growth. Plants that are young and actively growing ("vegetative") have more protein and energy and are richer in antioxidants. On the very best pasture, cattle gain weight almost as rapidly as they do in the artificial conditions of a feedlot. But if the plants are poorly managed and allowed to go to seed ("head out") or become woody ("lignify") they lose much of their food value and become less appealing to the cattle. The cattle grow more slowly, and the nutritional value of their meat declines as well.

The solution to keeping plants young and vigorous is to stock the pasture with just the right number of animals—not too many or too few—and then orchestrate their grazing so that they are eating grass at its optimum stage. To manage this feat, the Drakes have divided the pasture into smaller fenced areas called "paddocks." The animals are kept in a given paddock just long enough to crop all the plants down to about six inches in height. At this critical juncture, they are moved to an adjacent paddock and don't return until the grass has fully recovered.

This enlightened style of ranching is called "management-intensive grazing" and it promotes soil health and productivity. This is a marked improvement over letting cattle graze a large, undivided area of land. All too often, minimally managed cattle overgraze the land, not allowing time for the grass to rebound. As a result, barren areas appear that are vulnerable to wind and water erosion. Much of the western grassland has been overgrazed, causing significant environmental damage. In terms of environmental impact, management-intensive grazing is to unmanaged grazing what a solar-powered car is to a one-ton truck.

In terms of energy use, the differences between a pasture-based farm and a feedlot operation are even more dramatic. Most of our animals today, including cattle, are being "finished" in Concentrated Animal Feeding Operations, or CAFOs—corporate-owned, highly-mechanized, fuel-intensive factory farms where large numbers of animals are confined in a small amount of space. Old MacDonald did not have a CAFO. The cattle are raised outdoors in feedlots—large tracts of bare ground where the cattle stand around waiting to have their feed dumped into troughs. Managing one of these feedlots requires dozens of pieces of expensive gas-guzzling equipment. First, trucks are needed to haul the calves from the farms to the feedlot, which may be hundreds of miles away. Raising the corn and soybeans to feed the calves requires tillers, seed drillers, crop dusters, and combines. After harvest, the corn and soy are in constant transport, going from drying site to storehouse to processing plant and then to wholesalers and retailers for distribution. Finally, the feed is trucked to the feedlot, where it is doled out to the cattle on a daily basis by conveyer belts or trucks. It has been estimated that it takes a half a gallon of fuel to produce one pound of beef from a factory farm.[1]

In the feedlot, the cattle are confined to a small area and their manure builds up into huge mounds. The manure must be collected and deposited in manure lagoons—fetid ponds of water and manure—

or trucked to nearby fields. Because it costs money to transport the manure, it is often moved the shortest distance possible. As a consequence, the surrounding land can become overloaded with nutrients, polluting the soil and water.

When cows are raised on pasture, the use of fuel and equipment is minimal. To begin with, there is no need to transport the animals to the feedlots or the feed to the animals. The cattle stay on the farm until they're ready for market. To feed them, all you have to do is open the gate to an area of fresh pasture and step out of the way; grazing animals are highly motivated mowing machines. When the grass is sparse, you haul hay to the cattle in a pickup. Manure management is just as simple. The cattle spread their manure as they graze, part of nature's fuel economy. Because the manure is spread over a large area of land, it is a welcome source of organic fertilizer, not a "manure problem."

The Drakes like to tell people that their ranch is "solar powered." They see the pasture as a gigantic solar panel. The plants capture energy from the sun, draw carbon dioxide from the air, and siphon up minerals and water from the soil. Through the alchemy of photosynthesis, they transform these raw elements into a high-protein, high-fiber, vitamin-enriched food, ideally suited for grazing animals. Cows, sheep, and bison require only a few additional nutrients to thrive. The vitamin D that they need is produced automatically whenever the sun shines on their hides. The only other missing nutrients—vitamin K and the B vitamins—are manufactured by obliging bacteria that colonize their digestive tracts. Nature has worked out all the details.

As you continue your pasture walk, you are now close enough to see that dozens of chickens are sharing the field with the cattle and llamas. This is not a monoculture operation; it's a menagerie. The Drakes point out that the chickens are following behind the cattle and picking insect larva from the manure. As the birds peck and scratch, they quickly disperse the fresh piles, spreading the fertilizer more evenly. A manure pile can disappear with just a half hour of avian attention.

Weeks later, when the cattle revisit that particular paddock, new grass will be growing where the manure used to be, and there will be fewer flies to harass the cows.

Eleanor suggests that you sit down where you are and observe the cattle. The cattle may be domesticated, she explains, but they are still wary of humans, especially ones they don't know. You spot ten calves mingled with the herd. Most of the cows are intent on grazing, but a few are more vigilant and keep their eyes on you.

George explains that when they move the cattle from one paddock to the next, they herd them with subtle, strategic movements that are in tune with the animals' natural behaviors. Because they have mastered these techniques, the two of them can move the cattle by themselves without the need to ride horseback, whistle, wave their arms, circle lassos, crack whips, yell, or resort to a cattle prod. They can remain perfectly silent, keep their hands in their back pockets, and still move the animals where they want them to go.

As you walk slowly back to your car, the Drakes talk about when and why they left their jobs in the city, and how much they have learned in the past eight years. As you are about to leave, Eleanor runs into the house and comes back with a package of steaks. She wants you to sample the meat before you place a large order.

That evening, when you sit down to one of the grilled T-bone steaks, you realize you have a new meaning for the popular term "Value Meal." The value in this meat isn't that it is cheap or supersized. Rather, the meat was raised in a manner consistent with your *values*. You saw firsthand that the Drakes' farm is integrated with the natural environment, the animals are healthy and well cared for; the local ecosystem is being enriched and protected; and the Drakes are making a good living on the farm. This is one of those times when the food itself is the cause for celebration.

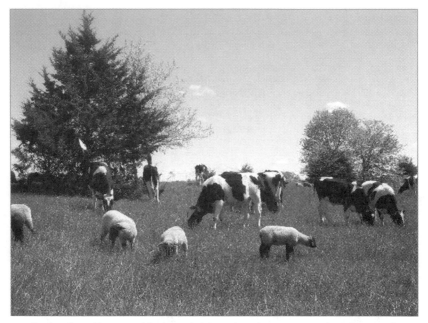

Schafer Farms Natural Meats, Jamesport, Missouri

Chapter 2

Back to Basics

For most people, the motivation to switch to grass-fed products is more than a wish for healthier food and a more humane way of raising animals. They also want cleaner, safer food. When they purchase a pound of conventional hamburger, they are worried that the meat might contain traces of hormones and pesticides, or bacteria that cause foodborne illness. Hamburger no longer seems safe.

Ten years ago, most people in this country were satisfied with the meat, eggs, and dairy products they found in the stores. As long as the food was USDA-inspected and reasonably priced, they found little to complain about. They also paid little attention to the way the animals were being raised. They viewed meat as something you bought at the supermarket that was wrapped in plastic on a Styrofoam tray. Few people knew that the animals that provided the food had been confined in crowded sheds and feedlots and treated with hormones, antibiotics, and other growth-promoting chemicals. Nor did they know that the animal industry had been taken over by a handful of conglomerates whose gigantic "factory farms" had all but replaced family farms. Bossy no longer grazed on green grass. She spent her days inside a building, alternating between eating grain, being milked, and lying down. Every two weeks she'd be injected with hormones to maintain a high level of milk production.

The public began to lose their complacency about factory farming in the early 1990s. First came the news that a growing number of people were being infected with a deadly form of E. coli bacteria. Most of the cases were traced to under-cooked hamburger. The most deadly outbreak occurred in 1993 in Seattle, Washington, when a fast-food chain sold hamburgers contaminated with E. coli that sickened an estimated 600 people. Some of the victims became very ill.

One hundred fifty were hospitalized, 28 required kidney dialysis, and 3 children died. Each passing year brought more outbreaks and more meat recalls. Meat safety became a major concern and remains so today.

Then along came "mad cow" disease, triggering an even deeper wave of anxiety. For about a decade, cattle in Great Britain and other European countries had been dying from a fatal brain disease called Bovine Spongiform Encephalopathy, BSE, commonly referred to as mad cow disease. This was distressing to European beef producers, but of little concern to consumers, especially those of us in the United States because it was all happening "over there." Then in 1995, a young British man died from a rare but fatal brain disease called Creutzfeldt-Jakob Disease, or CJD, that closely resembles BSE in cattle. CJD was not a new disease. But the British case was different. The victim was younger than usual, and his symptoms were atypical. As the months went by, more people were diagnosed with this new variant of CJD. By 2000, 84 people had died from the disease.

What was causing this horrific disease? Eventually, the story was revealed. The surge in mad cow disease was caused by a rarely discussed but widespread practice in the feedlot industry—feeding cattle to cattle. To the beef industry, turning meat scraps from cows into food for other cows was an efficient, cost-cutting measure. To the public, it was repellent.

But what was the connection between mad cow disease and Creutzfeldt-Jakob Disease in humans? A leading theory was that people got the disease when they ate portions of the brain or nervous tissue of cattle infected with BSE, most likely because those tissues had been mixed in with hamburger or sausage. Just a few bites of bangers or bratwurst could cause the bizarre disease to leap from cattle to people.

Now, for the first time, the livestock industry itself was being held up to scrutiny. It wasn't the cows that were mad—it was the cattle *industry*! Without announcing the fact, feedlot managers had been turning herbivores into cannibals, violating a natural barrier that had protected them from disease. What's more, this was not just another case of good meat being contaminated with bacteria: the meat *itself* was bad. No amount of hand washing or knife cleaning or cooking was going to get rid of the problem. How long had cattle been eating other cattle? What else were they being fed? Who was regulating their diets? What else was going on inside those cloistered factory farms?

It wasn't long before the public heard about another widespread but little known practice: most of the animals being raised in factory farms are being treated with synthetic hormones, low-level antibiotics, and chemicals for the primary purpose of speeding them to market. Our nation's cattle, chickens, turkeys, lambs, and dairy cows were on drugs.

Reeling from all these discoveries, some people stopped eating meat altogether. For these new vegetarians, avoiding meat was more an act of self-protection than a religious or moral issue. Soy was safer. Others switched to organic products. Organic certification gave them the assurance that the animals hadn't been treated with hormones or antibiotics and that their feed was pesticide-free. For the most part, it was the absence of "bad" things that drew people to organic meat and dairy products.

At the start of this century, consumers discovered another alternative to factory food—buying their meat, eggs, and dairy products from grass-based farmers. This was not just a step back in time. The farmers were using new management techniques, creating very high-quality products, and working hard to safeguard the environment. This was grandpa's farm, run by his studious, hardworking, principled, risk-taking grandchildren. And this new/old way of farming seemed a positive step into the 21st century.

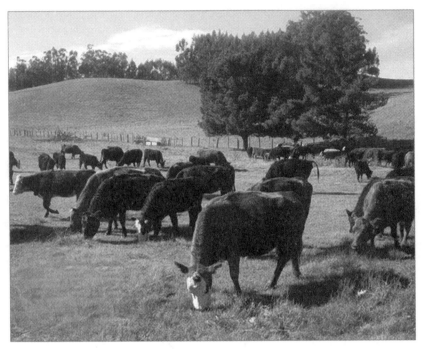

T.O. Cattle Company, San Juan Bautista, California

Chapter 3

Down on the Pharm

In the remaining chapters, I'm going to be describing the specific benefits you get from pasture-raised meat, eggs, and dairy products. In this chapter, I'm going to give you an insider's view of factory farming. I've learned that you can't fully appreciate grass-based farming until you know what it's replacing. I'm going to focus on just one part of the industry—poultry production. But the underlying premises apply to all CAFOs. Throughout the industry, the primary objective is to raise the animals as quickly as possible for the least amount of money in the least amount of space and with only minimal attention paid to the well-being of the animals or the workers. This draconian system is deemed necessary to "feed the world," assure corporate profitability, and satisfy the consumer demand for affordable food.

At the turn of the last century, most families in rural communities kept their own flock of laying hens. Old hens that had stopped laying became Sunday night's chicken and dumplings. People in the cities got their eggs from small-scale producers located in the nearby countryside. With each passing year, the number of poultry producers diminished, but the most dramatic change took place within the last decade. In the early 1990s, there were approximately 2,500 egg producers. There are fewer than 300 today. That's an 88 percent drop in just ten years. Our nation's mega-farms produce 73.8 billion eggs per year—246 million eggs per facility. This is not your grandmother's backyard flock.

Poultry CAFOs have dramatically altered the way eggs are produced, starting with the redesign of the birds themselves. Through selective breeding, "high merit" chickens have been created that lay phenomenal numbers of eggs each year. The common ancestor of our modern layers is the red jungle fowl of Southeast Asia that lays a few clutches of eggs each year. By the 1960s, selective breeding had transformed this ancestral bird into super-producing chickens that could lay 200 eggs per year. Today's best layers pump out 300 or more.

A rarely discussed flaw in this "more is better" strategy, is that chickens cannot produce 300 eggs a year without compromising their health. For example, no matter how much calcium is added to their diets, they cannot absorb enough to make 300 shells a year. Having no other option, their bodies leach calcium from their bones. By the end of their fleeting, 12-month laying life, most birds have porous or broken bones. This condition can progress to paralysis and a potentially fatal illness called "caged layer fatigue."

Another flaw in the system is the chickens have great difficulty generating enough fat to make 300 yolks. A consequence is that they develop fatty livers. The more eggs they lay, the more likely they will develop "fatty liver hemorrhagic syndrome," which causes them to bleed to death internally. Both of these physical problems can be traced directly to accelerated egg production.

In addition to changing the chickens themselves, poultry producers have been reducing the space allotted per bird. In today's CAFOs, laying hens are housed three to five to a cage, with only 50 to 60 square inches per bird. (For reference, a square foot is 144 square inches. Imagine two-and-a-half fully grown chickens squatting on a one-foot-square floor tile.) To keep the distressed birds from pecking at each other, their upper beaks are removed. In 2000, the McDonald's Corporation made headline news by requiring that their egg suppliers allot 72 square inches per chicken, which, according to careful research, provides enough room for all the birds in the cage to lie down at the same time. At least they no longer have to take shifts.

To anyone who has observed free-ranging chickens, the notion that 72 square inches of caged real estate is "humane treatment" is sheer lunacy. Birds raised on pasture are free to scratch for bugs, graze on grass, preen, chase dragon flies, and lie down with wings spread to capture the warmth of the sun. At night, they roost side-by-side in sisterly companionship.

But even though increasing a layer's living space to 72 square inches is a paltry improvement, conventional poultry growers are publicly begrudging the costs. They worry that those extra inches mean that the birds will move more freely, thus burning more calories and requiring more food. With easier access to the feeder, they also fear that the birds will spill more feed. The factory farm model may be efficient, but it has such a tight profit margin that there is almost no room to improve the welfare of the hens.

Conditions in the other half of the poultry industry—raising meat birds or "broilers"—are just as grim. As in the egg-laying industry, much of the focus has been on developing super chickens. In 1935, a typical broiler reached market size in five months. Our factory-farmed chickens hit the frying pan at six and a half weeks! Due to this breakneck rate of growth, their bones cannot provide enough infrastructure for their heavy-breasted bodies. The list of skeletal abnormalities in confined laying hens includes long bone distortion (bowed leg), tibial dyschondroplasia, rickets, kinky back, brittle bone disease, spraddled legs, infectious synovitis, viral arthritis, and foot pad dermatitis.

These painful conditions can be traced directly to modern breeding and feeding. A 1994 North Carolina study compared the incidence of bone problems in old-fashioned chickens with modern broilers.[1] One percent of the older breed developed skeletal problems. By contrast, 49 percent of the designer birds were afflicted—a design flaw in anyone's books.

Statistics tell only part of the story. You have to visit a broiler facility to get the full impact. In 2003 I had a chance to visit "Stacy and Bill Edwards," contract producers for a large east coast poultry conglomerate. (You'd recognize the name instantly.) In industry terms, the Edwards are in the "grow-out" business. This means that the company supplies the Edwards with chicks and chicken feed at regular intervals, and the Edwards supply the housing and labor. On a prearranged date, a company truck pulls into their driveway with 15,000 newly hatched yellow chicks. The chicks are deposited into a corner of the Edwards' 300-foot-long metal shed. The chicks stay in the shed on the same bedding for just over six weeks, at which time they have grown large enough to create a living, wall-to-wall feather carpet. They are now ready for market, and the company sends out a crew of "chicken catchers" to take them to the processing facility. On a typical day, a crew of eight captures between 40,000 to 50,000 chickens from several different farms. The day is done when all of the birds have been rounded up. A common complaint of the workers is that they are not always paid for their overtime.

I arrived at the Edwards' the day before the chicken catchers were due to arrive. I'd never toured a confinement poultry operation before, so I had no idea what to expect. I parked my car close to the long metal shed so that I could take a quick look around. As I walked toward the building, I expected to hear a cacophony. Eerily, I heard nothing but the hum of machinery. Fans? The only tip-off to the fact that there were 15,000 birds inside was the stench of ammonia that wafted out of the vents. It was breathtaking.

Stacy came out to greet me, explaining that Bill had yet to come home from his full-time day job. Like most contract growers, raising chickens provided only a portion of their income. She opened the door at the end of the shed and let us into a small room separated from the birds. She handed me a pair of rubber boots and suggested that I take some deep breaths. She warned that I wasn't going to feel like breathing when she opened the door. She pointed to half a dozen 5-gallon buckets filled with dead birds. Her 11-year-old twin boys had collected them that afternoon. The boys' daily "farm chore" was to get rid of the carcasses before the other birds had cannibalized them. ("John-Boy, go collect the dead chickens before you go out and play.")

Stacy told me that most of the chickens had died from "ascites," a pneumonia-like condition that afflicts birds that grow so quickly that their lungs and hearts can't keep pace. In the final stage of the disease, the circulation to the birds' lungs is so poor that they drown in their own juices. In essence, the birds are given the death sentence for over-achieving. An estimated 2 to 4.7 percent of all broilers die in this manner. Eight billion broilers are being raised each year in this country, so even if the two percent death rate is used, the death toll from ascites alone is 160 million birds a year.

Given the extent of this carnage, one might think that ascites is extremely hard to prevent. Not so. It's purely a matter of economics. The simplest and most direct way to prevent ascites is to slow the growth rate of the birds. You can do this in a number of ways, including using a slower-growing strain of bird, lowering the protein content of the feed, or by removing the growth-promoting additives. But no one is considering these options. Even though ascites costs the industry an estimated $1 billion per year, the amount of money gained by the rapid growth of the surviving chickens more than offsets the losses.

Stacy opened the inner door, and I was overwhelmed by the sight of so many living creatures crammed into one place. I couldn't take a step without first scooting birds out of the way. To my surprise, the chickens were not milling around but lying quietly on the soiled litter. The reason they were so subdued, Stacy explained, is that in accordance with company policy, they kept the lights dim so that the birds wouldn't become agitated or cannibalistic. Except for the time the chickens spent feeding and drinking, they sat quietly in their own waste, waiting for their dawn appointment with the chicken catchers.

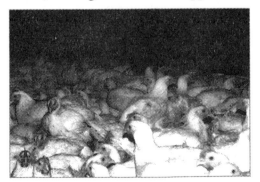

As Stacy had warned me, it was getting difficult to breathe. My lungs were working just fine, but I had a strong aversion to filling them with ammonia fumes. From my reading, I had learned that anyone who spends just three hours inside a confinement poultry operation will start to wheeze, cough, and develop lung inflammations.

I couldn't help wondering how the birds were being affected by the fumes. Their heads were only inches away from their excrement. From reading poultry science journals, I had learned that chickens that are exposed to 50 parts per million of ammonia, which can happen at the end of a growing cycle, develop burns on their breasts, their eyes become lopsided and watery, their faces swell, and they develop eye lesions that can lead to blindness. Some contract producers are unable to monitor ammonia levels effectively during a grow-out because they have become desensitized to the odor. They don't realize there is a problem until the birds show obvious signs of distress.

Reducing ammonia levels in a poultry shed, like preventing ascites, is a simple matter. You can make life more bearable for the birds by replacing all the litter between grow-outs, allocating fewer birds per shed, or running the ventilation fans night and day. The reason the industry hasn't made these changes is that it would lower company earnings beyond the comfort level of the owners and managers.

As my eyes adapted to the dim light, I could see that many of the birds were panting. I hadn't expected this, given the fact it was only 45 degrees outside. Then I realized that the birds themselves were generating the heat. There were so many of them, and they were packed so closely together that the indoor temperature must have been 80 degrees or more. Stacy told me that if the fans were to go off on a summer day, the birds would die from their own waste heat in a matter of hours. This was her worst nightmare. Like all contract growers, she and her husband had installed generators to take over during a power outage. But that meant that one of them had to be on the premises 24-hours a day to turn them on.

"Have you ever eaten any of the chickens?" I asked.

"We never have," she said. "We have to use the company feed, and they won't tell us what's in it. One thing we do know is that it contains arsenic, which is why we've been told to wear gloves when we handle the feed."

Arsenic? Later, when I researched the use of arsenic in the poultry industry, I learned that it helps control a few diseases, but its main function is stimulate the birds' appetites. Arsenic is also used in the swine industry, with the FDA's seal of approval. The practice is so widespread that arsenic from animal waste is polluting our land and water. The top poultry-producing region of the country is the "Delmarva Peninsula," which includes parts of Delaware, Maryland, and Virginia. Each year, 600 million chickens produce more than 1.5 billion kilograms of manure. This translates into a load of 44 to 110 thousand pounds of arsenic.

Stacy volunteered that the feed contained antibiotics as well. When animals are raised in close quarters under stressful conditions— in other words in a factory farm—disease spreads quickly. To help prevent disease and simultaneously speed the growth of the animals, the birds are given a steady diet of low-level antibiotics. According to a comprehensive report issued by the Union of Concerned Scientists in January 2001, "…livestock producers in the United States use 24.6 million pounds of antimicrobials [antibiotics] for nontherapeutic purposes….Seventy percent of all antibiotics in the U.S. are fed to pigs, poultry and cattle for reasons other than treating disease. The majority of such medicines are 'medically important'—that is, identical, or nearly so to antibiotics used for humans." When large numbers of animals are given a particular antibiotic, strains of bacteria develop that resist the drug. When we humans become infected with the resistant bacteria, there is one less antibiotic to fight it.

Alarmingly, the percentage of salmonella bacteria that has developed resistance to as many as five different antibiotics has increased from less than one percent in 1980 to 34 percent in 1996. In a 1997 study, scientists isolated bacteria from chicken eggs and exposed them to a wide range of antibiotics.[2] They detected resistant strains of some of our most common foodborne bacteria, including Staphylococcus aureus, Enterococcus faecalis, E. coli, Enterobacter cloacae, Pseudomonas stutzeri, and Citrobacter freundii—a veritable army of superbugs! Many believe it's only a matter of time before these resistant bacteria cause widespread health problems.

After spending only 20 minutes inside the shed, I told Stacey that I was ready to leave. I'd seen too many panting, pecked upon, and dying birds, and inhaled too much ammonia and fecal dust. When we walked outside, I felt as though we were ascending from Hades.

A few days later when I showed some of the pictures I'd taken to a group of friends, they reacted with disgust. At first, they refused to believe that the boneless chicken breasts that they popped into their supermarket carts came from birds like the ones I was showing them. I assured them that this was indeed the case. In fact, the next time they went to the supermarket, they might buy meat from one of these very birds. A chicken that looks stressed and abused on the day of slaughter looks just fine when cut into uniform pieces and wrapped with plastic. The words on the label are targeted to calm any concerns one might have about the meat. This chicken is "Fresh, All-Natural, and Locally Grown!"

My visit with Stacey reinforced my commitment to buy only pasture-raised poultry. Factory-raised chicken is enticingly cheap, but a steep toll is paid by the birds, the contract growers, the chicken catchers, and the land. The poultry that I serve to family and friends comes from a farmer who runs his chickens with his cattle. At night, the birds roost in a portable hut where they are safe from predators. During the day, they roam the pasture. Their meat is more flavorful and juicy than commercial chicken. No mushy, watery, tasteless flesh. Also, the bones are remarkably strong. It takes effort to make a wish on a wishbone.

Chapter 4

Exploring the Feed/Food Connection

Many people who shop for food at their local grass-based farms make the trip because they want to bring home the healthiest possible food. Although they appreciate the many other benefits of grassfarming, their main interest is in getting the most wholesome and nutritious meat, eggs, and dairy products they can buy.

The livestock industry and most health authorities have been slow to acknowledge the health benefits of pasture-raised products. They still cling to the belief that the way animals are raised and what they are fed makes no difference to their meat, milk, or eggs. This reluctance to acknowledge any connection between what animals are fed and what we eat is surprising, given the fact that neon signs have been highlighting the link for decades. For example, it is a well known within the livestock industry that our cattle are being fed a long list of ingredients in addition to soy and corn. These rarely talked about supplements are referred to as "by-product feedstuff." This broad category includes: 1) recycled human food, such as stale candy, pizza, potato chips, brewery wastes, and hamburger buns; 2) parts of our fruits and vegetables that we don't eat, such as orange rinds, beet pulp, and carrot tops; and 3) stuff you don't want to know about including chicken manure, chicken feathers, newsprint, cardboard, and "aerobically digested" municipal garbage.

Chicken manure is a very popular feedstuff for cattle and sheep in the south and the central east coast because those areas are home to so many chicken factories. Chicken manure costs from $15 to $45 a ton compared with $125 a ton for alfalfa—a welcome savings.

Few would argue that chicken manure has the same food value as high quality pasture, or that candy bars are as nutritious as clover. But, for a variety of reasons, no one has been measuring the effect that by-product feedstuff has on our food. I have searched diligently, but have yet to find a study that shows how feeding manure to animals changes the nutritional value of their meat, milk, eggs, and dairy products. The underlying belief is that eggs are eggs, meat is meat, and milk is milk, no matter what the animals are fed. The concept "garbage in, garbage out" has yet to be applied to modern animal agriculture.

For me, one study epitomizes this "anything goes" mentality. In the mid-1990s, a team of animal researchers decided to investigate the possibility of feeding stale chewing gum—still in its wrappers!—to cattle.[1] Wonder of wonders, the experts concluded that the bubblegum diet produced a net benefit—at least for the producers. I quote: "These data indicate that gum and its packaging material can safely replace at least 30% of growing and finishing diets without impairing feedlot performance or carcass merit." In other words, fatten cattle on bubblegum and aluminum foil wrappers, and you'll save money without slowing down the growth rate of the cattle or lowering the quality grade of their meat. Such a deal!

With a nod to public safety, the researchers *did* run tests to determine how much aluminum was being deposited in the various organs of the cattle. Not to worry. The aluminum content was "within normal expected ranges." But no one bothered to take the next critical step and measure the nutritional value of the meat. Beef is beef is beef. When I first read the study, I assumed that no one would actually *feed* bubblegum to their animals, despite the recommendation of the researchers. Then an animal scientist drove me by a gum factory in upstate New York where dairy farmers picked up truckloads of free chewing gum.

One of the essential underpinnings of our factory farm system is the belief that our livestock can be fed anything that is cheap and available without changing the food on our table. So what if the system stresses the animals, spawns antibiotic-resistant bacteria, pollutes the air and water, and is leading to the demise of small family farms?

As long as the CAFOs produce large quantities of nutritious food at a reasonable price, the system is working. End of discussion.

It's time to set the record straight. Factory farms are producing nutritionally inferior food. And feeding our animals manure, garbage, and gum is only part of the problem. *The greatest upheaval comes from the simple fact that the animals are eating less grass and more grain.* This may come as a surprise to people who grew up thinking that the terms "grain-fed" and "corn-fed" are indicators of quality. But as you will see, switching animals from grass to grain lowers the vitamin content of their products, diminishes the amount of good fats, and boosts overall fat and calories. The extent of these nutritional differences depends on the type of animal and exactly what it is fed. I will provide these details in the next few chapters. But first, I want to take a step back and give you the big picture.

Less Fat. One of the main reasons animals are fed large amounts of grain is that they grow fatter faster. Grain is a more concentrated form of energy than grass and provides more starch and calories. The net result of a high grain diet is fattier beef, lamb, bison, and chicken. Products from feedlot animals have from one-third to three times more fat than animals raised on pasture. Most grass-fed meat is so lean that it has about the same amount of fat as wild game or a skinless chicken breast.[2] (See graph on the following page.)

Fewer Calories. Because most grass-fed products are leaner than grain-fed products, they also have fewer calories. A six-ounce beef loin from a grass-fed cow may have 92 fewer calories than a six-ounce loin from a grain-fed cow. If you eat a typical amount of beef per year, which in the United States is about 67 pounds, switching to grass-fed beef will save you 16,642 calories a year. All things being equal, you will lose 9½ pounds in two years without having to change your eating habits or use an ounce of willpower.

Nine and a half pounds may not sound like all that much, but it's more with than most people lose on structured weight loss programs. For example, according to a recent study, a typical dieter following

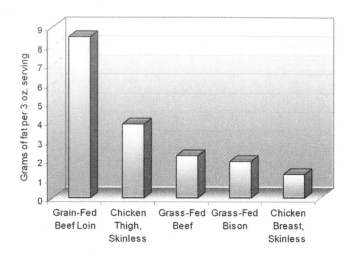

Meat from grass-fed animals is much lower in total fat than grain-fed animals, and even lower than skinless chicken thighs.
J Animal Science (2002). 80(5):1202-11.

the Weight Watcher's Program loses 6.4 pounds in two years, a modest weight loss that requires eating fewer calories, attending meetings, using a point system, and making food substitutions. It appears to be easier to lose weight by changing the diet of our animals than by trying to change our own!

More Omega-3s. Meat, dairy products, and eggs from grass-fed animals offer you more omega-3 fatty acids then products from grain-fed animals. The health benefits of this "good" fat are becoming well known. Careful research shows that people who are low in omega-3s have a higher risk of a host of diseases and conditions including cancer, depression, obesity, diabetes, arthritis, allergies, asthma, and dementia. Men and women low in omega-3s are also more likely to have high blood pressure and an irregular heartbeat.[3] Ominously, women whose diets contain the least omega-3s are twice as likely to die from a heart attack or stroke.[4]

One reason these ailments are so prevalent in the United States is that our diet, like most western diets, is abnormally low in omega-3s. Twenty percent of Americans have levels so low that they defy detection.[5] One reason we are so deprived is that we eat relatively small amounts of fish, walnuts, flaxseeds, and dark green leafy vegetables—foods that are good sources of these healthy fats.

But more than people realize, taking our animals off pasture has contributed to the deficiency. Buy your food from a grass-based producer and it will contain 2 to 10 times more omega-3 fatty acids than food from the grocery store.[6] The explanation is straightforward. Omega-3 fatty acids originate in green plants. Whether this healthy fat is in a trout, a bottle of canola oil, a handful of walnuts, or a roast from a grass-fed steer, it was created by plants or algae. For example, the reason that fish are rich in omega-3s is that little fish dine on omega-3 rich algae and phytoplankton. They, in turn, are gobbled up by bigger fish, which carry the good fat up the food chain. Grass is an especially rich source of omega-3s. As a direct result, animals that graze on grass have more omega-3s in their meat, eggs, and dairy products. Animals, too, are what they eat.

Keeping Omega-6s and Omega-3s in Balance. Compared with grass, grain is very low in omega-3 fatty acids and high in omega-6 fatty acids, a competing type of fat. Both of these fats are essential for our health, which is why they are called "Essential Fatty Acids" or EFAs. As a general rule, however, omega-3s and omega-6s have opposite effects on your body. For example, foods high in omega-6 fatty acids promote blood clotting, while foods high in omega-3 fatty acids slow it down. Both properties are essential. After a serious injury, blood clots need to form immediately or you risk bleeding to death. But the rest of the time, your blood needs to flow freely. If your diet contains too many clot-promoting omega-6s and too few clot-busting omega-3s, there is the risk that an errant clot will develop inside your arteries, cut off the blood supply to your heart or brain, and trigger a heart attack or stroke. For optimum health, you need the right mix or ratio of EFAs.

What is the right ratio? Health experts are still hotly debating the issue, but most experts agree that an ideal diet should have no more than four times as many omega-6 fatty acids as omega-3s.[7] Some people peg the ratio as low as one-to-one because this is the type of diet eaten by our ancestors who survived on wild plants and game.[8] Nature's banquet is nutritionally correct. This is why tribes of hunter-gatherers were able to survive and thrive without taking a class in fatty acid chemistry. We would still have a one-to-one ratio today if we lived in the wilderness and gathered our own food.

One of the ways we upset this essential balance is by taking our animals off omega-3 rich grass and switching them to omega-6 rich grain. A cow raised on grass has a healthy omega-6 to omega-3 ratio ranging from three-to-one to less than one-to-one. A cow raised on grain has an unhealthy ratio ranging from five-to-one to as high as fourteen-to-one.[9] When we put our animals back on grass, we help bring our entire diet back into balance.

Conjugated Linoleic Acid. Ruminants are animals with multi-chambered stomachs that allow them to get maximum food value from grass and other greens that are high in cellulose—a type of starch that humans cannot digest. All members of the ruminant family, including cattle, dairy cows, goats, bison, sheep, deer, and elk, can survive and thrive by grazing pasture or browsing leaves and brush.

Ruminants share another trait as well: their products contain a newly discovered "good" fat called "conjugated linoleic acid," or CLA. When the animals are raised exclusively on grass, their meat and dairy products offer two to five times more CLA than animals raised on large amounts of grain.[10] (Monogasts—animals with single stomachs such as pigs and poultry—have little or no CLA, even if they are raised on pasture.)

CLA shows promise of helping us fight two deadly diseases—cancer and cardiovascular disease. A great many studies have shown that CLA fights cancer in lab animals. In a recent study, for example, feeding rats small amounts of the same type of CLA found in ruminants shrank their mammary tumors by 45 percent.[11]

It's too early to say whether or not CLA will fight cancer in humans as well. A well-designed cancer study costs hundreds of millions of dollars and may take decades to produce meaningful results. But there are indications that CLA might lower the risk of breast cancer. A 1996 study of 4,697 women revealed that the more full fat milk in a woman's diet—thus the more CLA—the lower her risk of breast cancer. The women who drank the most milk had a 60 percent lower risk than those who drank the least. A more direct connection comes from an Irish study. Scientists extracted CLA from the milk of grass-fed cows and added very small amounts (20 parts per million) to human breast cancer cells growing in culture. By the eighth day, the CLA had killed 93 percent of the cells.[12] Lastly, a group of Finnish researchers found that women who consumed the most CLA in their diets had a 60 percent lower risk of breast cancer than those who consumed the least.[13] Although this is too little data to make a valid health claim about CLA and breast cancer, the signs are pointing in the right direction.

There are also encouraging signs that CLA might help people with clogged arteries. Once again, most of the evidence comes from animal studies. In a 1994 study, researchers gave CLA to rabbits that had the classic signs of coronary heart disease.[14] The CLA reduced the amount of fatty deposits inside their arteries by 30 percent, actually reversing the condition. CLA from grass-fed products may help humans in a similar way. In a 2002 study, a group of healthy volunteers were given CLA supplements.[15] The CLA lowered a type of cholesterol that is a high risk factor for heart disease. The researchers concluded that "this study confirms that some of the cardio-protective effects of CLA that were shown in animal studies are relevant to man."

So far, you've seen that products from animals raised on pasture ✓ have less fat, fewer calories, more omega-3 fatty acids, fewer omega-6 fatty acids, and, in the case of ruminants, more CLA. In the next chapters you will see that they also have a bonus supply of vitamins A,

E, folic acid, and beta-carotene. When all the nutritional differences between grain-fed and grass-fed products are totaled up, the superiority of grass-fed products is undeniable.

How did we allow the food value of our animal products to be changed this significantly? Wasn't anyone paying attention? Although it's tempting, I don't see the diminished nutritional value of our food to be the result of evil wrongdoers. It's just agribusiness as usual. The problem is that animal production is treated exactly like automobile production: do everything you can to lower costs and maximize profits. If this involves stressing the animals, giving them a totally artificial diet, and implanting them with hormones—so be it. The bottom line is that you have increased company profits. This mindset works as long as you view animals as inanimate objects and disregard the fact that people are eating the products that come off your assembly line.

There's another reason for the loss of nutritional content in our food: arrogance. Many people in the health and food industries assume that whatever information they have at any given time is sufficient to allow them to make radical changes to our food supply without cause for concern. For example, our ruminants were taken off pasture 50 years before anyone knew that grass-fed animals produced more CLA than grain-fed animals or even that CLA had any health benefits at all. The policy is to act now and deal with the consequences later. The idea that we should study natural systems before we alter them is alien to industrial agriculture. Consumers who are uncomfortable with the steady advance of food technology are at risk of being labeled "reactionary" or "uninformed."

A British study published thirty years ago drives this point home.[16] At the time of the study, people were growing uneasy about the egg-laying business. Twenty years earlier, half of all laying hens had been raised outdoors on pasture. By 1970, 94 percent of them were confined to indoor cages. As the investigators began their research they noted: "It is a popular view that eggs produced by modern intensive farming methods are nutritionally inferior or less wholesome than those produced by traditional methods." Like consumers today who are worried about the implications of genetically modified food, the Brits were worried about the wholesale changes in poultry production.

Was the public reacting to change itself? To answer the question, the British scientists scrutinized eggs from free-range and factory-raised chickens. After careful analysis, they discovered only two differences: eggs from the pastured hens had 50 percent more folic acid and 60 percent more vitamin B12 than eggs from factory-farmed hens.

These findings were downplayed, however, because comparatively little was known about these two vitamins. In fact, no daily minimum requirement had been set for either of them. Today, the medical literature boasts thousands of studies about the key roles they play. We now know, for example, that vitamin B12 is essential for nerve function, the production of red blood cells, and the manufacture of DNA—the genetic material in all cells. Folic acid (folate) is necessary for the healthy development of the fetus and may also help prevent heart disease, depression, cervical cancer, colon cancer, and prostate cancer. Many Americans are deficient in folic acid, so in 1992 the government mandated that the nutrient be added to all our cereals, pasta, flour, and corn meal. Little did we know that confining our layers to indoor cages was helping to create this deficiency.

The British assessment of the eggs was hampered by another knowledge gap: no one knew about the importance of omega-3 fatty acids. It wasn't until 1982 that the omega-3s were recognized as essential for health, and research in the field did not begin in earnest until the mid-1980s. Not knowing better, the British team did not even bother to measure the amount of omega-3s in the eggs. From later research, we know that eggs from free-foraging hens can contain up to 10 times more omega-3s than eggs from confined birds.[17] Not privy to this fact, the team came to the following conclusion: "The main finding of this survey was that there was very little difference in the chemical composition of the eggs...." Due to their lack of knowledge, raising hens in cages and feeding them an industrial-strength diet was deemed A-OK.

The parable of the eggs holds true for the entirety of modern livestock production. The factory model had replaced Nature's model before anyone understood the full impact on human health. But that's no excuse for continuing agribusiness as usual. It's time to learn from past mistakes and return to healthier modes of production. This isn't a simple turning back to 19th century farming. To create sufficient amounts of pasture-raised foods at a reasonable cost—without making undue compromises—will require the best minds in animal science aided by state-of-the-art technology. Having disassembled the natural system, science will have to rebuild it.

Some of that work is now underway. Researchers in the field of sustainable agriculture have found a number of ways to make pasture-based farming more efficient while staying true to the natural model. For instance, one group found that cattle grow faster if they are fed hay that is harvested in the afternoon, which is the time of day when the grass has the highest sugar content. Surprisingly, the amount of the resulting gain is equivalent to that produced by hormone implants. A second group found that calves grow more quickly if they are kept with their mothers for an extra few months. And this prolonged suckling does not interfere with the cows' ability to produce another calf the following year. If the research community conducts more studies such as these, we will be headed back in the right direction.

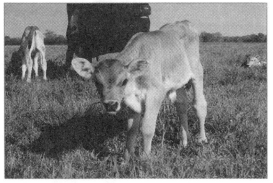

Jako, Inc.,
Hutchinson, Kansas

Chapter 5

Grass-Fed Beef: One of the Healthiest Foods on the Menu

Red meat has gotten a bad rap in recent decades. Anyone who is overweight, has a serious health problem, or simply wants to have a healthy diet is advised to cut back on red meat and eat more chicken or fish. The underlying assumption is that all red meat is the same. In truth, grass-fed beef is healthier for you than grain-fed beef, and, surprise, surprise, it may be even better for you than chicken. The color of the meat isn't the problem. It's what the animals are fed.

Let's take a closer look at the health benefits of grass-fed beef. Like all beef, it's a good to excellent source of high-quality protein, iron, zinc, selenium, phosphorous, and the B-complex vitamins. But it is superior to grain-fed beef in a number of key ways. As I mentioned in the previous chapter, it is lower in fat and calories and higher in omega-3 fatty acids and CLA. These differences alone justify a switch to pasture-raised beef.

Vitamin E. There's more. Grass-fed beef provides more vitamins as well. When cattle are raised on pasture, their meat gives you more vitamin E. Vitamin E is one of our most important antioxidants because it protects us from free radicals, boosts our immunity, and may lower our risk of coronary heart disease. Grass-fed animals have more vitamin E than grain-fed animals for a very good reason: grass and clover have 20 times more of this nutrient than corn or soy, the main ingredients in a feedlot diet. Grazing cattle consume as much as 1,000 IU of vitamin E each day, 10 times more than found in a typical feedlot diet.[1] One study determined that there is from three to six times more vitamin E in grass-fed meat than feedlot beef.[2] The more vitamin E in the feed, the more vitamin E in the meat, and the more that

✓   gets passed on to us. We are what our animals eat.

Carotenoids. Grass-fed beef is higher in a number of antioxidants in the carotenoid family, including lutein (LOO-teen), zeaxanthin, (ZE-uh-zan-thin) and the more familiar beta-carotene.

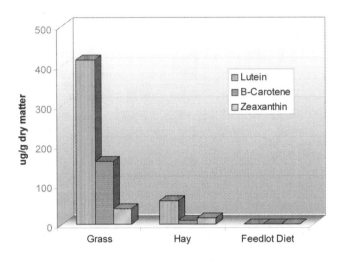

Grass has more carotenoids than hay or a typical feedlot diet
J Animal Science (2003). 81:360-367.

Fresh pasture offers hundreds of times more of these nutrients than a standard feedlot diet.[3] As a result, grass-fed meat has up to four times more beta-carotene than conventional feedlot meat. You can see the difference by looking at the color of the fat. The more carotenoids, the more golden the color. Fat from feedlot meat is stark white. Fat from grass-fed meat ranges from a creamy hue to almost yellow, depending on the quality of the grass and the age and breed of the animal. Unfortunately, people who have been eating grain-fed beef all of their lives are not accustomed to seeing any hint of color in the fat. According to a report issued by the University of California, "Discounts on [beef] of up to 20 cents per pound can occur due to the public's conditioned preference to the white fat produced from grain feeds that are lower in beta carotene."[4]

In countries where animals are still being raised on grass, *white* fat is viewed with suspicion. A chef from Argentina remarked, "Looking at the fat of a USDA Choice steak is like looking at the face of a dead man." People who have switched to grass-fed beef would agree.

The benefits of eating a diet rich in carotenoids include a lower risk of cataracts and macular degeneration, the leading cause of blindness in the western world. Also, in a recent study, women with the highest levels of beta-carotene in their diets had half the risk of breast cancer as those with the lowest.[5]

When you add up the score card between grass-fed and grain-fed beef, grass-fed beef wins hands down. The more naturally raised meat has:

- Less overall fat
- Fewer calories
- More omega-3 fatty acids
- A healthier ratio of omega-6 to omega-3 fatty acids
- More CLA
- More vitamin E
- More beta-carotene

Given all these benefits, a steak from a cow raised on pasture is even healthier for you than a chicken breast—the white meat that health authorities are so quick to recommend. The steak has about the same amount of total fat, making it an equally good choice for a heart-healthy diet, but it has more omega-3s, as you can see by the following graph. (See next page.)

What's more it has less cholesterol than chicken and more than four times more CLA.[6] Move over chicken. Make room for grass-fed beef!

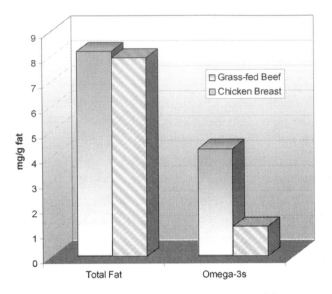

Grass-fed beef has the same amount of fat
as a chicken breast but more omega-3s
J Animal Science (2002). 8(5):1202-11.

Chapter 6

Super Healthy Milk

Tour the dairy section of your supermarket and you will see an array of cartons picturing black and white spotted cows grazing on bright green grass. In most instances, this is deceptive advertising. The majority of our cows are being fed grain in confinement dairies. They eat dried hay instead of grass, and the ground they stand on is either concrete or a blend of dirt and manure.

Cows are kept in confinement and fed a high-grain diet so they will produce the maximum amount of milk. To speed things along, they are injected with hormones on a biweekly basis. The system works. In the 1940s, a good milk cow produced around 4,500 pounds of milk per year. Today's cows produce 20,000 pounds or more per year—more than a four-fold increase. A few super producers exceed 30,000 pounds per year. One record-breaking Holstein has produced enough milk to fill nine semi-tanker loads, or about one million glasses of milk. And she's still going.

In all of the euphoria over this flood of milk, the dairy industry has swept aside one central fact: milk, butter, and cheese from grain-fed cows are less nutritious than those from grass-fed cows. Once again, quality has been sacrificed to quantity.

A major benefit of milk from grass-fed cows is that it contains more CLA. This discovery was made in the mid-1990s by Tilak Dhiman, a dairy researcher at Utah State University. At that time, animal scientists around the globe were looking for ways to produce high-CLA milk from cows fed a typical feedlot diet. Among other things, they supplemented the cows with chemicals called "ionophores," rapeseed meal, extruded oil seeds, recycled restaurant grease, and vegetable oil. While these experiments were going on, Dhiman got the idea to test the milk of 100 percent grass-fed cows. To everyone's surprise, the milk from grazing cows had "500 percent

✓ more conjugated linoleic acid in their milk fat than cows fed typical dairy diets."[1] This difference was so large and so unexpected that Dhiman had to repeat the test several times before his colleagues accepted the results. Returning cows to their native diet turned out to be the most effective strategy of all.

✓   In addition to giving you more CLA, milk from pastured cows offers more omega-3 fatty acids and fewer omega-6 fatty acids, resulting in a healthy ratio of one-to-one. As the following chart shows, the more grain in a cow's diet, the less balanced the EFA ratio.

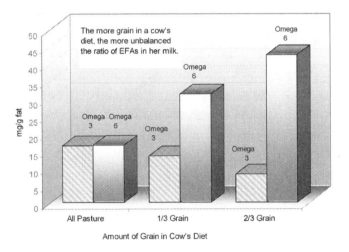

J Dairy Science (1999). 10:2146-56.

Keep Bossy on grass and her milk will have more beta-carotene, vitamin A, and vitamin E as well.[2] These extra vitamins show up in all her dairy products, including milk, butter, cheese, yogurt, and ice cream. This vitamin bonus comes, in part, from the fact that fresh pasture itself has more of these nutrients than grain or hay.

But there's another, less obvious reason for the greater concentration of vitamins. A cow gets a set amount of vitamins from her food, and the more milk she produces, the fewer vitamins she has for each glass of milk. Milk from a high-producing, grain-fed cow, is a watered down version of the real thing. According to researchers who have studied this phenomenon: "It follows that breeding and management systems that focus solely on increasing milk and milk fat yield will result in a steady dilution of vitamins and antioxidants."[3] A clear example of more is less.

As with grass-fed meat, you can tell that dairy products from pastured cows are rich in beta-carotene by the color of the fat. Serve cheese or butter from a grass-based dairy and everyone will notice the difference. People who were born after the 1960s may think the food has been helped along by Yellow Dye #22. To them, a white stick of butter looks more natural.

In search of healthier dairy products, many consumers choose organically certified milk, butter, and cheese. Organic milk is superior to ordinary milk because the cows are not treated with artificial hormones or antibiotics, more attention is paid to their comfort, and their feed is free of pesticides. But most organic milk is less nutritious than grass-fed milk. The reason is that most organic dairies feed their cows significant amounts of grain. Although the grain is raised organically, it is grain nonetheless. Because the cows are eating more grain and less grass, their milk has less CLA, fewer omega-3s, less vitamin E, and more omega-6s. For the healthiest milk, cows need more than an organic diet; they need their original diet.*

---

*   *Some organic dairy producers keep a significant number of their cows on pasture during the spring and summer, enhancing the nutritional value of the milk. Others raise their cows in confinement year-round. Check with a dairy directly to learn more about their practices. Also, be aware that some grass-based dairies are organically certified, the best of both worlds!*

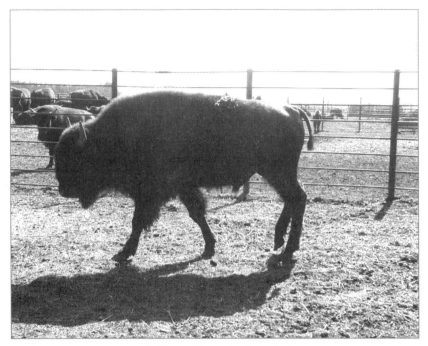

Solitary Bison in Feedlot

Chapter 7

Grass-Fed Bison, Lamb, and Pork

T he first pasture-based farm I ever visited was a Texas bison ranch. At the time, I thought that all bison were grazing on prairie grasses. In fact, I recommended bison to anyone who wanted to eat meat that was similar to wild game. But my hosts told me that most of these magnificent beasts are now being fattened on grain in feedlots, just like cattle. The reason? The bison need to be fat enough "to meet the requirements of the consumer."

Once again, the bison are at the mercy of humans. First, they were slaughtered almost to extinction for their skins and horns. Now, they are being penned up and treated like domestic cattle. Shortly after visiting the grass-based bison ranch, I toured a bison feedlot in Nebraska. It was a sweltering July day, and I couldn't shake the feeling that the animals had been sentenced to a maximum security prison.

Feeding grain to bison makes even less sense than feeding grain to cattle. Our modern breeds of cattle are the result of centuries of selective breeding that has succeeded in calming their dispositions and increasing their ability to pack on the fat. As a result, they are relatively easy to handle in captivity and bulk up quickly in the feedlot. Today's bison, however, are just as wild as they were hundreds of thousands of years ago, making it much more difficult to keep them confined. Unlike cattle, they will jump fences and break through most man-made barriers.

What troubles the bison industry the most is that the animals are slow to fatten up in the feedlot, the most expensive part of the production cycle. The reason the bison resist gaining weight is that their bodies remain adapted to life on the prairie. During the winter months, when the prairie grasses are dormant or covered with snow, their appetites decline and their metabolic rates slow down significantly. There's no point in being hungry and burning excess fuel when there's so little food. Over the winter, they may lose ten percent of their body weight. When spring arrives and the grass rebounds, however, their metabolism fires up once again and they became avid grazers. Within weeks, they have made up for the winter loss and begun to lay down additional fat—a built-in survival strategy known as "compensatory gain." The growth rate of the bison and the natural growth cycle of the prairie grasses are in perfect harmony, a synergism that came from eons of co-evolution.

This synergism is now being pried apart. Many bison producers select their breeding stock from those rare animals that put on weight year-round, a trait that is a liability in the wild. Other bison managers select their stock from animals that weigh the most at weaning. The bigger the calf, the more meat is produced in a given amount of time. These unnatural selections are not without consequences. The incidence of difficult bison births is on the rise. Two of the main reasons are that the cows are overly fat or the calves are disproportionately large. Breeding animals for one or two specific traits will always have unwanted consequences.

Yet more innovations are underway. A common practice is to speed the growth of the bison with light therapy. In the winter months, bison producers mount banks of bright lights over the feedlots. In much the same way that light therapy devices ease winter depression in humans, these lights alter the biorhythm of the bison, tricking their bodies into thinking it's spring. As a result, they eat more steadily throughout the winter and lay down more fat.

Grass-based bison ranchers reject this "bigger, faster, better" mentality. One producer, Jan Beckert, told me that she focused her energy on improving the pasture, not the bison. "I think that the bison are pretty highly evolved just as they are." On *www.eatwild.com*, you will find dozens of other ranchers who share this hands-off philosophy.

When you choose grass-fed bison, you are doing more than supporting ranchers who let bison be bison. You are also getting more nutritional benefits. As is true for grass-fed beef, meat from pasture-raised bison has less overall fat, fewer omega-6 fatty acids, and more CLA and omega-3s than grain-fed bison. Grass-fed bison boast a very healthy EFA ratio of two-to-one. Bison that have been penned and grained have an EFA ratio as high as seven-to-one.[1]

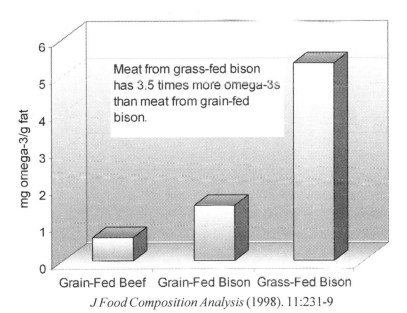

J Food Composition Analysis (1998). 11:231-9

To make matters worse, grain-feeding also raises the cholesterol content of bison meat as you can see by the graph on the next page.

The overall trend in bison production is to produce meat that is more like feedlot beef. Producers who raise their bison on grain are going to lose those customers who are searching for alternatives to grain-fed beef.

Grass-Fed Lamb. Fifty years ago, there were 56 million sheep being raised on American farms. Today, there are fewer than seven million, an eighth of the former number. In 1945, lamb comprised four percent of our total meat consumption. Now it's a mere 0.6 percent.

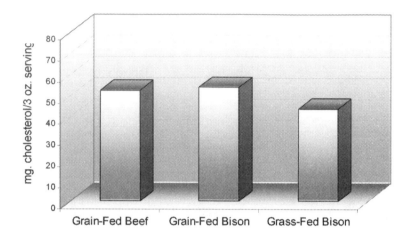

Meat from grain-fed bison has more cholesterol than meat from grass-fed bison, and as much as meat from grain-fed beef.
J Animal Science (2002). 80:1202-11

That amounts to only one pound of lamb per person per year. One reason people are avoiding lamb is that they think it's too fat. Most of our lambs are now being fattened on grain, which can make their meat quiver with fat. According to meat merchandiser Marty Gardner, "The U.S. buyer wants to buy pasture-fed lamb that is free of antibiotics and less fatty…"

Presently, most of the grass-fed lamb in this country is being imported from New Zealand and Australia, partly due to its lower cost. Raising sheep on pasture is less expensive than raising them on grain, especially in countries that have spent decades perfecting grass-based production. But imported grass-fed lamb is superior to American grain-fed lamb in a number of ways, according to Rosemary Mucklow, executive director of the U.S. National Meat Association. "Imports fill the need for tenderness, when American [grain-fed] lamb tends to be tough and gamey…"

In past years, we were importing so much lamb from Down

Under that the U.S. government enacted a nine percent tariff to protect our grain-based sheep industry. The tariff was declared illegal by the World Trade Association and eliminated in 2001. But before the government removed the tariff, it set aside $47 million dollars to purchase grain-fed American lamb, hoping to shore up the struggling industry.

In another attempt to support the conventional U.S. sheep industry, animal scientists have been looking for ways to lower the cost of production. A number of strategies have worked, including feeding lambs recycled newsprint treated with hydrogen chloride for up to 40 percent of their diets, and feeding them a combination of hog and poultry manure—good sources of phosphorous and magnesium.[2]

There is an alternative to the current strategies of: 1) blocking the import of grass-fed lamb, 2) subsidizing U.S. grain-based producers, and 3) feeding lambs newsprint and manure: encourage more farmers to raise their sheep on pasture. Pasture-raised lamb is leaner, more tender, more flavorful, costs less to produce, and is in high demand.

It is also more nutritious. In fact, grass-fed lamb has more omega-3 fatty acids and CLA than either grass-fed beef or bison.[3] Furthermore, it is rich in lutein, a member of the carotenoid family that helps protect eye health.[4] To top it all off, grass-fed lamb has a low EFA ratio of one-to-one compared with eight-to-one for grain-fed lamb.[5] Raising lambs on pasture is a winning package.

Pastured Pigs. The trend in hog production, like the trend in the overall livestock industry, is to replace independent, farmer-owned hog farms with monolithic, corporate-owned confinement facilities. Consolidating hog production has serious repercussions. For every $5 million in investment, between 40 to 45 new jobs are created. But each new hog factory puts an estimated 126 independent hog farmers out of business, resulting in a net job loss.[6] What's more, hog factories buy most of their supplies from within the company, bypassing local suppliers and further undermining the local economy.

People who live close to a hog factory have more immediate worries. A North Carolina survey of 155 people determined that the closer people lived to a confinement hog operation, the more health problems they had, including more headaches, runny noses, sore throats, coughing, diarrhea, and burning eyes.

As you might expect, the people with the most health problems are those who work inside the factories. According to an Iowa State University report, workers in swine buildings are exposed to dangerously high levels of dust, ammonia, carbon dioxide, and other gasses. "It is common to have swine buildings with ... [dust] concentrations high enough that one is unable to see clearly across a 100-foot room. Nearly 70 percent of the workers experience one or more symptoms of respiratory illness or irritation."[7] They also are prone to hypersensitivity pneumonitis and are at risk of hydrogen sulfide poisoning. Workers in hog factories have more job-related health problems than workers in any other confinement operation.

Too bad no one heeded the advice of a 1965 study that compared raising pigs on pasture with raising them indoors on concrete. As is true for most confinement operations, the pigs on concrete gained weight faster and were fed for a shorter period of time. But it cost more per pound to raise them because the pasture-raised pigs got a significant amount of their nourishment from grass. The confinement-raised pigs also "showed signs of stiffness and lameness, especially as they reached market weights." The quality of their meat suffered as well. It was "softer in finish than those raised on pasture. These conditions could result in a reduction in selling price." The conclusion of the report? "This trial shows that good pasture can account for a substantial saving in feed costs. This saving, plus the absence of lameness and a firmer finish of the meat, favors the use of pasture where possible. These advantages may become even more important where rations are not adequately balanced for protein, vitamins, and minerals because pasture can supply many of these factors." This report should be dusted off and assigned to students in animal agriculture.

People who live close to pasture-based hog operations appreciate the fact that they produce very little odor. Researchers at Texas Tech University have a demonstration pasture-based hog operation. When the site was being designed, the university staff assumed it would smell as bad as a typical confinement operation. John McGlone, who was in charge of the project, told his colleagues that it wouldn't smell, but no one believed him. "I had them out there in the fields a year after we started, and they couldn't believe it. It doesn't smell." Workers in the hog industry would appreciate the clean air even more.

In addition to all these benefits, pork from pigs raised on pasture is more nutritious than pork from factory farms. The meat has more vitamin E and more omega-3 fatty acids.[8] Future studies are likely to add to this list.

In taste comparisons, many people choose pastured pork over grain-fed pork. The traditional hog industry has put so much emphasis on producing low-fat pork that many people find it dry and flavorless. Pork from pastured pigs tends to be more flavorful and juicy, bringing to mind the pork chops and roasts of decades ago.

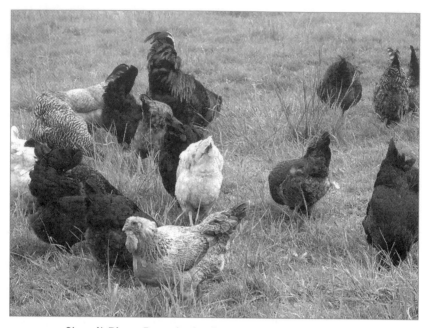

Skagit River Ranch, Sedro Woolley, Washington

Chapter 8

Free-Living Poultry

R uminants and pigs are not the only animals you will find happily grazing on pasture-based farms. Chickens, turkeys, ducks, and geese are busy foraging as well. Unlike ruminants, however, they are not designed to survive on pasture alone. They need some form of high quality protein as well, such as insects or a mixture of grains and legumes. But pastured chickens will get as much as 30 percent of their nutritional needs from insects, grass, clover, and other greens; turkeys, ducks, and geese are more eager grazers and can glean as much as 50 percent of their calories from pasture. As a result of all this greenery, their meat and eggs have higher amounts of omega-3 fatty acids, vitamin E, vitamin A, folic acid, and carotenoids as compared to similar grain-fed products.

Dr. Artemis Simopoulos, co-author of *The Omega Diet* and an international authority on health and nutrition, was the first person to document that eggs from free-roaming hens are good sources of omega-3s. While visiting her family's farm in Greece, she noticed that the chickens spent much of their time foraging on wild greens, in particular a common weed called purslane. In earlier research, she had found that purslane is very high in omega-3s. She wondered—would the nutritional content of the purslane be reflected in their eggs? To find out, she hard-boiled half a dozen eggs and took them back to the United States for analysis. The lab results showed that the Greek eggs had ten times more omega-3 fatty acids than eggs purchased from the supermarket. What's more, their EFA ratio was an ideal one-to-one. The supermarket eggs had a very unbalanced ratio of twenty-to-one, consistent with the hens' high-grain, no-greens diet.[1]

Barbara Gorski, a pasture-based poultry producer, secured a small federal grant to test the nutritional content of her eggs and broilers.[2] Compared with eggs from caged birds, the eggs from her pastured flock had 10 percent less fat, 40 percent more vitamin A, and 400 percent more omega-3 fatty acids. An unexpected finding is that the eggs also had 34 percent less cholesterol (160 mg. per egg versus the customary 214.) This finding is noteworthy because poultry scientists have struggled for decades to find ways to lower the cholesterol content of eggs. Among other things, they have fed hens a long list of pharmaceutical drugs and chemicals, such as cupric sulfate pentahydrate, cholesterol, O-acyltransferase, lovastatin, colestipol, and di-(2-ethylhexyl) phthalate—with little or no change in the eggs' cholesterol levels. Now we know that letting hens loose to forage on greens and insects does the trick. Once again, nature's original plan is proving to be the superior plan.

Barbara got an equally positive report about her broiler chickens. Compared with commercial birds, their meat had 21 percent less total fat, 30 percent less saturated fat, and 28 percent fewer calories. The breast meat was so lean that it qualified for the USDA designation of "fat free." It also had 50 percent more vitamin A and 100 percent more omega-3s. Health care providers take note: consider recommending *pastured* poultry products.

Meat from pastured poultry is not only healthier, it tastes better as well. In a blind taste test of ordinary and free-range Thanksgiving turkeys, *The New York Times* food editors chose a free-range bird as their number one choice. They reported that the meat was flavorful and juicy and had a tender but meaty texture. Owners of fine restaurants concur. When you order chicken or turkey at an upscale restaurant, the meat is likely to come from a free-range bird.

People who raise pastured layers tell me that their customers recognize the superiority of their eggs instantly. They don't need to read studies or listen to the food critics to know that the eggs are better for them. A woman who sells her eggs at a farmer's market reports, "All I have to do is crack open one of our eggs and an ordinary egg. One look, and people line up to buy ours. The yolks are almost orange! We have to ration the eggs to have enough for our regular customers."

Once people start eating eggs from pastured hens, it's hard for them to go back. Joel Salatin, a recognized master of pasture-based production, tells a story about one of his more devoted customers. She called him one day to ask if he had any eggs for sale. She had company coming for breakfast the next day, and she couldn't bear the thought of serving ordinary eggs. Joel said he was sorry, but he only had a half dozen eggs. The women said, "That's okay! I'll take whatever you have! I'm leaving right now, and I'll be there in an hour and a half." She was willing to make a 200-mile round trip just to pick up a half dozen eggs.

"Customer retention" is a continual battle for food producers. A large company may spend millions of dollars to establish brand recognition. Then it pays millions more to make sure its products are displayed on the most favorable shelves in the supermarket. But consumers keep switching brands, nonetheless, usually because of cost or convenience. There is so little brand loyalty that the sale of most food products will go down if they are moved to a lower shelf. Shoppers find it too much trouble to bend at the waist to pick them up. Factory food creates fickle shoppers.

At the present time, there are hundreds of pasture-based poultry producers throughout the country. And they never seem to have enough eggs to go around. But this is just a fraction of one percent of the gigantic poultry industry. Will pastured poultry and eggs ever gain a significant share of the market?

It's certainly possible, as has been demonstrated by the "Label Rouge" phenomenon in France. Forty years ago, Label Rouge was a grassroots movement led by a handful of visionary farmers who were protesting the trend toward factory farming. Their goal was to develop a method of raising livestock that protected the environment, respected the animals, allowed farmers to make a reasonable income, and, being Frenchmen, produced the very highest quality food. These goals are shared by most of the pastured poultry producers in the

United States.

Today, Label Rouge chickens commandeer 30 percent of the market, even though they cost *twice* as much as conventionally raised birds. French consumers are also happy to pay more for Label Rouge ham, sausage, eggs, rabbit, and cheese products.

It's enlightening to learn about the production standards for raising Label Rouge broilers. Once the birds reach six weeks of age and are fully feathered, they must have free access to the outdoors from 9 a.m. until dusk. Each bird is guaranteed at least 22 square *feet* of range land—not a square foot of floor space. Their feed cannot contain animal products, antibiotics, or growth stimulants. Beak and toe trimming are not allowed. And, in stark contrast to the American "bigger, faster" mentality, the birds must grow slowly enough that they do not develop growth-related health problems. In fact, the standards specify that the broilers cannot be sold until they are 81 days old—a month later than our fast-track American broilers. Label Rouge is a shining example of the international Slow Food movement. More and more people around the world are discovering that the way to optimal health and maximum pleasure is to pay more for your food and eat less of it.

Will pasture-raised poultry, lamb, bison, pigs, and cattle find such a warm welcome in the United States? Admittedly, the "pay more, eat less" philosophy is a harder sell in the land of 44-ounce Super Big Gulps and half-pound candy bars. But throughout the country, tens of thousands of people are now spending their grocery money on pasture-raised products. By making this choice, they are supporting local farmers, enhancing the welfare of the animals, protecting the environment, and bringing home the highest quality eggs, meat, and dairy products. What's more, they're spreading the good news about grassfarming one friend at a time.

Go Grass!

Chapter 9

Where Do You Find It?
How Do You Cook It?

A t the present time, there may be as many as a thousand pas ture-based farmers who sell their food directly to the public through on-farm sales, Internet websites, or at farmers' markets. Some of the larger farms sell to retailers and restaurants as well. If you live in a large metropolitan area, especially on the east or west coast, you may find pastured products at a local store. If a nearby store doesn't carry them, or if you prefer to buy your food directly from a farmer, you will need to do some hunting and gathering.

If you are searching for a local supplier, I recommend that you visit my website, *www.eatwild.com*. It contains an updated, state-by-state listing of suppliers. No third-party certification is available at this time, but the farmers listed on the site pledge that they meet the following criteria:

- Raise ruminant animals on forage only. (Mineral supplements and kelp, etc. are OK.)
- Raise dairy animals on pasture with no grain, or minimal amounts of grain. (They must specify if the animals are fed any grain, concentrate, or silage other than grass silage.)
- Raise poultry on high-quality pasture (free-range, day-range, or in moveable cages) supplemented with grain and other wholesome ingredients.
- Raise pigs and rabbits on high-quality pasture, supplemented with grain and other wholesome ingredients.
- Practice holistic and/or environmentally sound management.
- Demonstrate active concern for animal welfare.
- Use no growth hormones or artificial growth enhancers.
- Use antibiotics only when an animal is sick or injured.
- Organic certification is desirable, but not essential.

You can look for grass-fed products at your local farmers' market and natural foods stores. In some locations, you can join a grass-fed products buyer's club. (You place your order along with other members and either the supplier brings the food to a central location or someone in your group goes to the farm to pick it up. If you can't find a buyer's club, consider starting one, even if you start with only one or two other members.)

Ideally, you will find a supplier in your local area. When you buy locally, you can see first hand how the animals are raised. Producers who don't want to give you a tour may have something to hide. (I have yet to be invited to tour a feedlot or conventional slaughter facility. In fact, I was even instructed to leave the premises when I was taking pictures of a feedlot from my car on a county road.) Buying locally also eliminates the environmental toll caused by long-distance shipping, supports local farmers and the local economy, and helps preserve nearby agricultural land.

If you are unable to find a supplier close to you, you can have products shipped to you. As a general rule, only the larger farms take mail orders. Ordering through the mail increases your overall costs considerably, but the quality of the meat shouldn't suffer. Frozen meat packed in lots of ice or dry ice and shipped via overnight delivery should arrive at your door frozen solid. If not, most grassfarmers will refund your money. (Note: Some farmers won't ship their products in the summer months because they can't guarantee their meat will arrive in good condition.)

When you find a potential supplier or products at a local store, make sure you're getting the real McCoy. As of this printing, there are no universally accepted terms or standard for pasture-based food, although efforts to establish them are underway. At present, products are marketed using a bewildering array of terms. These include "salad bar beef," "free-range," "grass-fed," "pasture-finished," "grass-finished," "pasture-ized," "100 percent grass-fed," "naturally raised," "range-fed," and "New Zealand-Style." How do you figure out what these mean?

"Pasture-finished," "grass-finished," and "100 percent grass-fed" are among the most reliable terms when it comes to describing ruminants. Most ruminants are raised on grass for the first few months of their lives, so technically, even feedlot beef could be called "grass-fed" or "free-range." Some less than candid producers use these terms, even though their animals spend the last months of their lives in a feedlot or on the farm being fattened on grain and other supplements. It is likely that you will have to ask the producer or retailer about production methods. If you have a difficult time getting a straight answer, chances are the terms are just marketing ploys. Keep in mind that terms such as "all-natural," "wholesome," "naturally raised," and "like the food from Grandma's farm," tell you nothing about how the animals are raised or what they were fed.

For the best quality product, look for animals that have been raised on pasture all of their lives. But there is a middle ground between raising animals in a feedlot and raising them on grass alone— I call this category "pasture-raised." To qualify for the term, the animals must be actively grazing whenever grass is available and must not be treated with low-level antibiotics, artificial hormones, or other growth promoters. What distinguishes "pasture-raised" from "pasture-finished" is that the animals can be supplemented with non-grass products whenever high quality pasture is not available. Ideally, the supplemental feed is made up of ingredients such as flaxseeds, full-fat canola meal, some types of soy, and fish meal that enhance the nutritional value of meat and dairy products, not diminish it.

Raising animals on pasture and giving them a limited amount of other types of feed is superior to raising them in feedlots. The animals are less stressed and less prone to disease, and there is little negative impact on the environment. In addition, local farmland is preserved, and the farmer—not a large corporation—reaps the profits. But the gold standard will always be "all grass, all the time." This method produces food that is better for us, keeps animals on their native diet, and uses pasture to its maximum potential.

Some pasture-based farms are organically certified, which means that the pasture is raised according to strict organic guidelines and that the farmers have certified that their animals are not treated with feed antibiotics, synthetic hormones, or other chemicals. Most grass-based farms do not have this designation. Some don't qualify because they apply nitrogen fertilizers to their pasture or medicate their animals to eliminate worms and other parasites. Some grassfarmers are unable to locate an organically certified butcher or a sufficient supply of organic grain. The realities of the marketplace hold back others. Many hog and poultry producers, for example, find that organic grain is too expensive to allow them to make a profit.

Nonetheless, most pasture-based farmers follow the organic model as closely as possible. Very few use insecticides, herbicides, genetically-modified grain, metabolic modifiers, by-product feedstuff, routine antibiotics, or artificial hormones. Just because farmers lack organic certification don't assume they practice agribusiness as usual. Ask.

A New Way to Shop. Once you've selected a supplier with high-quality products, you may not find that the food is available just when you want it. Few grassfarmers manipulate their animals to produce out-of-season or to force their growth. For example, most grass-fed cattle, bison, and lamb are butchered at only specific times of the year, times that are dictated by local climate conditions. In some parts of the country, animals are slaughtered in the fall before the grass goes dormant. In other areas, animals are slaughtered in the late spring before the summer drought sets in. This is inconvenient if you are shopping for a fresh leg of grass-fed lamb the day before Easter, or T-bone steaks for your Fourth of July picnic. To have what you want when you want it, you may have to buy a year's worth of meat in October and store it in your freezer or a commercial locker. Some producers advise you to sign up for your free-range Thanksgiving turkey a year ahead of time. Also, some of the better known farms—

especially those that have been featured in the media—may have more customers than they can handle. You will be referred to another producer or put on a waiting list.

Picking up Your Order. Few small-scale grassfarmers have enough freezer or refrigerator space to keep large quantities of meat chilled or frozen. If you are buying directly from a farmer, you may be asked to pick up your order on a specific date. If the broilers are butchered on Tuesday morning, for instance, you may need to retrieve them by 6 p.m. that evening. Combining orders with a friend, family member, or buying club gives you more flexibility.

Some of these inconveniences reflect the fledgling state of the grassfarming industry. Every year, more farms are coming online and offer more of the amenities we've come to expect. But some "inconveniences" are inherent in the grassfarming process itself. Our desire to have fresh meat every day of the year does not mesh with the growing cycle of the grass or the natural breeding cycle of the animals. One of the reasons that we have embraced factory farming is that the food is always available when we want it. To have the most nutritious, environmentally-friendly food, we may have to change the way we shop.

Buying Meat for Your Freezer. When you make the transition to grass-fed meat, dairy products, and poultry, you may be buying large quantities of food and storing it in a freezer.

If you are buying a quarter, half, or whole animal, you pay a set price per pound, usually based on the "hanging weight"—the weight of the meat after the animal has been butchered but before it is divided into individual cuts. The amount you take home will be 25 to 35 percent less than the hanging weight due to trimming and boning. The net cost of the meat varies from farm to farm, but if you order meat in sufficient quantity, it is likely to cost only slightly more than ordinary supermarket meat. Some of the larger farms offer smaller packages of assorted cuts such as a 20-pound "grill pack" or a 15-pound "stew pack." The meat will be frozen, but you can store it in a small freezer.

To decide how much to buy, ask yourself how much meat your household will eat in the next six months. The typical adult eats 67 pounds of beef per year. Once you've decided on the total amount to buy, the supplier will present you with a "cutting list" and ask you to specify exactly how you want the meat cut up. Do you want more roasts or more hamburger? How thick do you want your steaks?

Having gone through this process for a number of years, I have learned to throw myself on the mercy of the producers. They know far better than I do how to divide up the meat. Except for asking for thicker steaks than usual and making sure I get my share of the "innards," I just tell them, "Give me your standard cut."

The following charts show the typical yield from a hind or a front quarter of beef. Many grassfarmers also offer a "split half." This is a quarter of beef that contains cuts from both the front and back quarters. The back quarter is considered more desirable, so offering cuts from both ends is a good way to lower the cost to consumers and utilize all the meat. Typically, beef quarters take up about four cubic feet of freezer space, which is about two average-sized shelves.

Yield from a Typical Hind Quarter of Beef (144 pounds)

Cut	Pounds
Round Steak	27.0
Rump Roast	9.9
Porterhouse, T-bone and Club Steaks	15.3
Sirloin Steak	24.9
Flank Steak	1.5
Lean Trim	21.0
Kidneys	0.9
Waste (fat, bone, shrinkage)	43.5
Total Hind Quarter	144.0

Yield from a Typical Front Quarter of Beef (156 pounds)

Cut	Pounds
Rib Roast	18.3
Blade Chuck Roast	26.7
Arm Chuck Roast (boneless)	17.4
Brisket (boneless)	6.3
Lean Trim	49.2
Waste (fat, bone, shrinkage)	38.1
Total Front Quarter	156.0

Poultry Products. When you shop for pastured poultry products, be on the lookout for pale imitations. "Free-range" and "organic" eggs, chickens, and turkeys are now widely available, and they command a premium price. But these labels do not guarantee that the birds have seen the light of day or nibbled a blade of grass. To qualify as "free-range," a bird has to only have *access* to the outdoors. The area outside the shed may be a mixture of dirt and chicken manure. Sunbathing is not the same as foraging.

Be wary of other misleading terminology as well. Chickens described as "uncaged" are likely to be spending their time milling around with 10,000 other birds in a crowded shed. Not being locked in cages may increase their comfort somewhat, but their meat and eggs will be no better for you than products from caged birds.

"Natural" is one of the most deceptive words in the food lexicon. The term has nothing to do with the way the animals are raised. According to the United States Department of Agriculture (USDA), any meat can be called "natural" or "all-natural" as long as it's been minimally processed and does not contain any artificial ingredients. Under this limited definition, even factory chickens can be described as healthy and natural, as the following comment from a marketer from Tyson Farms illustrates: "The leading national brands are just as natural as free range chickens. Most commercially grown chickens are fed only the highest quality grains, vitamins and minerals, in a controlled environment, to ensure a healthy, all natural product."

Is Grass-Fed Meat Tender? Pastured pork, lamb, and poultry are always tender, partly because the animals are harvested at an early age. Meat from grass-fed bison and cattle, however, can have varying degrees of tenderness, just like grain-fed meat.

What makes meat tender? Most people assume that the amount of marbling in beef or bison determines its tenderness: the fatter the meat, the more tender it's likely to be. They also assume that because grass-fed meat can be very lean, that it will be tough. In reality, marbling accounts for only 10 percent of the variability in meat tenderness. Genetics accounts for at least 30 percent. The rest of the variability is due to such factors as the location of the cut (loin or shoulder, for example), the age and sex of the animal, and the stress level of the animal prior to slaughter.[1] Many grassfarmers take great pains to maximize these "tenderness factors." Others do not. If you're not happy with the quality of the meat from a particular farm, shop around.

Tenderness can also be increased after the animal is butchered. This can be accomplished by: 1) mechanical alteration; 2) marinating; or 3) dry-aging. Mechanical alteration includes the pounding or grinding that produces pre-tenderized Swiss steaks, cutlets, or hamburger. Marinating is typically done at home, and consists of soaking the meat in an acidic liquid such as wine, lemon juice, or vinegar. In dry-aging, the whole carcass is held at a temperature just above freezing for one week or more. This practice intensifies the flavor of the meat and makes it more tender.

Dry-aging is generally not used in the conventional meat industry because it is time consuming and requires a lot of space. Unless otherwise noted, the meat you purchase at the supermarket has been "wet-aged," which means that it has been aged for several days in plastic. Most pasture-based producers go to the added trouble and expense to dry-age their meat to give you a premium product.

Cooking Grass-Fed Meat. Some grass-fed meat now on the market is every bit as tender as grain-fed meat and can be cooked in the same manner. Most grass-fed meat, however, requires special cooking techniques—especially the leaner cuts. Fat serves as an insulator. When meat has little fat, heat is conducted more quickly and can toughen the protein. To keep grass-fed meat tender, cook it more slowly and at lower temperatures. If you're broiling a grass-fed steak, for instance, place it farther away from the heating element or coals and cook it for a longer period of time. But don't cook it too long! Even the most tender cut of meat will become dry and tough if you overdo it. Steaks are best served medium to rare. The lower the finishing temperature, the more tender the meat will be. If you like your meat well done, don't grill it. Cook it with moist heat at a low temperature for a longer period of time.

Less tender cuts of meat such as a chuck steak or arm roast always need to be cooked slowly with moist heat. The crockpot I hauled out of the attic works just fine for grass-fed meat. If you're concerned about cooking grass-fed products, consider ordering hamburger or manually tenderized meat. This way you can savor the rich flavor of the meat without worrying about how to cook it. One thing you'll notice is that a pound of raw meat yields almost a pound of cooked meat—your burgers won't shrink on the grill.

Maintaining the Quality of Frozen Meat. If you are buying a large quantity of meat for your freezer, take steps to retain its high quality. Salting meat prior to freezing shortens its storage life, but coating it with herbs and spices (without salt) extends it. Rosemary and thyme are good herbs to use because they are potent antioxidants and excel at keeping the meat fresh.

If you are freezing several pieces of meat in the same pckage, separate the meat with double sheets of wax paper to make them easier to separate while thawing.

Meat will keep indefinitely at zero degrees Fahrenheit or below, but the flavor and texture of the meat will suffer over time. Air is the culprit. It dries out the meat and causes freezer burn—those brownish, dry patches. Freezer burn does not make the meat unsafe to eat, but it does alter its taste and appearance. The best way to protect the meat from air is to vacuum pack it in freezer-grade plastic bags. You can do it yourself or ask the butcher to do it.

If you order a large amount of fresh meat, such as a quarter or side of beef, you will not able to freeze it rapidly enough in a standard home freezer. The rule of thumb is to freeze no more than five percent of the capacity of your freezer at any one time. Slow freezing creates large ice crystals. During thawing, the crystals damage the cells, causing the meat to drip and lose much of its juice. It's better to have the meat flash frozen before you bring it home.

The most common way to wrap the meat is in butcher paper, freezer foil, freezer-grade plastic bags, or freezer-quality plastic wrap. (When using butcher paper, the shiny side goes next to the meat.) To maintain the high quality of the meat, remove as much air as possible. When using plastic bags, squeeze out the air and seal with twists or rubber bands. If you are using other types of packaging, wrap the meat tightly and tape the seams to keep out the air. Label all packages with the date, type of meat, cut, and quantity.

There are three safe ways to thaw meat: in the refrigerator; wrapped in a plastic bag and submerged in a sink or pan of cold water; or in the microwave. Thawing meat at room temperature warms the outside of the meat before the inside is completely thawed, allowing bacteria on the outside to multiply.

FARM RECIPES

For Grass-Fed Beef, Bison, Venison, Lamb, Veal, Pork, Poultry, and Eggs

BEEF RECIPES

SWEET GRASS FARM'S
PILGRIM POT ROAST

3 to 4 pound beef chuck roast
3 tablespoons flour
5 tablespoons shortening, butter, or bacon fat
1 teaspoon salt
$^1/_8$ teaspoon pepper
1 cup onion, chopped
¼ cup prepared horseradish
½ cup whole berry cranberry sauce
4 whole cloves
6 to 8 serving size potatoes
6 to 8 serving size carrots

Combine flour, salt, and pepper and dredge meat in the mixture. Brown the meat in the fat in a heavy pot with a tight fitting lid. After browning, add spices, cranberry, and horseradish. Cover tightly and cook very slowly for 2½ to 3 hours. Add vegetables, cook until tender.

Serve sliced on large platter with the vegetables and pass the gravy from the juice. Thicken gravy if necessary.

Wendy Gornick
Vernon, New York
wgornick@born.com

BURGUNDY PASTURE BEEF'S
FLAMBÉ ROAST

This is very simple and makes a wonderful broth—you add no liquid but the brandy. A bone adds richness to the broth, but a boneless roast works as well.

3 to 4 pound roast, bone in or boneless, preferably chuck roast
1 tablespoon olive oil
1 onion, coarsely chopped
2 ribs celery, coarsely chopped
1 cup small fresh mushrooms, preferably a dark, hearty mushroom
½ cup (or more!) brandy, cognac, or bourbon
2 to 3 leafy celery tops
1 fresh bay leaf
Fresh cracked pepper

If frozen, thaw roast and pat dry. Rub with fresh cracked pepper. In a Dutch oven, brown the roast well on all sides in olive oil. You do not need to have the stove on high heat, be patient and make sure you get a good "brown" on the roast. Remove roast to platter.

Sauté vegetables in the Dutch oven until semi-soft, then remove from heat. Set vegetables aside in a bowl. Place roast back in Dutch oven and pour brandy over it. Immediately light the brandy on fire and wait until fire goes out (shake the pan to burn off all the alcohol). Return vegetables to the pot along with celery tops and bay leaf. Cover pot and place in pre-heated 225–degree oven. Cook until fork tender, about 3 to 4 hours. Time will vary depending on the size of the roast. Salt the roast as desired after cooking or at serving.

Jon and Wendy Taggart
Grandview, Texas
www.burgundypasturebeef.com

RIVER RUN FARM'S
MARINATED GARLIC CHUCK ROAST

3 to 3 ½ pound boneless grass-fed beef chuck roast
   (you can also use rump or bottom round)
½ cup strong coffee
¼ cup soy sauce
¼ cup Yoshida's Original Gourmet Sauce
1 tablespoon dry sherry
1 tablespoon Worcestershire sauce
1 tablespoon red wine vinegar
½ teaspoon ginger
1 large onion, finely chopped
Garlic, about 1 whole bulb

Peel garlic and sliver part of it. Cut slits in meat with small sharp knife. Insert slivered garlic deep into slits all over the roast. Mince remaining garlic and mix with all ingredients, pour over roast. Marinate in refrigerator for at least 12 hours, turning several times.

Remove meat from marinade and broil meat in oven, or cook on grill. (I cook on a rotisserie.) Baste frequently with marinade. Cook to desired doneness. Best served medium-rare and thinly sliced. Serves 6 to 7.

James and Ellen Girt
Clatskanie, Oregon
info@riverrunfarm.com
www.riverrunfarm.com

SWEET GRASS FARM'S
TASTY STUFFED FLANK STEAK

2 to 3 pound flank steak

Stuffing:
½ cup oil , butter, or bacon fat
2 ½ cups bread cut into ¼–inch
  cubes
1 pound lean ground beef
2 eggs
1 onion, chopped
½ celery rib, chopped
2 cloves garlic, peeled and minced
2 tablespoons parsley, chopped
½ teaspoon salt
½ teaspoon pepper
¼ teaspoon crushed thyme or savory

> *Flank is fibrous and will be tough if not cut against the grain. However, properly prepared, flank is tasty and juicy. Slice thinly, like London broil.*
> *—Wendy Gornick*

Pull off the thin silver skin on one side and the fatter skin on the other side. Trim off excess fat at the end. Keeping the flank flat with one hand, cut into it lengthwise with a small, sharp paring knife to make a pocket for the stuffing. Lift up the upper "lip" and cut, keeping your blade horizontal. Be careful not to come out at either end. Cut deeper into the steak, but do not cut through to the other side. If you accidentally cut through the flank, slice a thin piece off an end where it won't affect the pocket and use it to plug the hole; the stuffing will keep it in place.

Brown the bread in the fat. Combine the remaining ingredients in a large bowl and then add bread cubes, mixing in lightly to avoid making a mush. Stuff the flank steak, tie the roast, salt and pepper all around.

You will need the following ingredients for braising:

2 tablespoons oil, butter, or bacon fat
1 medium carrot, diced
1 onion, chopped
2 bay leaves
1 tomato, about 1 cup coarsely chopped
1 teaspoon thyme leaves
1 cup water or stock
1 cup dry red wine
2 tablespoons arrowroot or corn starch
¼ cup cold water
Salt and pepper to taste

You will need a deep, heavy casserole with a cover. Heat the fat and brown the stuffed flank on all sides. Add the carrot, onion, bay leaves, tomato, and thyme and cook over moderate heat, uncovered, for 5 minutes. Add the water or stock and wine, bring to a boil, cover and braise on very low heat on top of the stove, or in a 300–degree pre-heated oven for 1½ hours. Lift meat to a platter, remove strings, and keep warm while making the sauce.

Remove most of the fat from the surface of the braising liquid. Mix the arrowroot or corn starch with the water and then stir into the braising liquid. Bring to a boil and cook, stirring constantly, until the sauce thickens slightly. Add salt and pepper to taste.

Wendy Gornick
Vernon, New York
wgornick@born.com

MISTY RIDGE FARM'S
CROCKPOT NO BOTHER ROAST

There is nothing as simple and delicious to prepare as a roast—with a crockpot.

Place frozen beef roast in crockpot. Add two cups of water Simmer about 4 hours on high heat, then switch to low heat.

About 90 minutes before serving, add potatoes, carrots, celery, onions, or other vegetables to your liking. Season with your favorite herbs. Turn up the heat to high. Add water only if needed.

Serve the most tender and delicious beef you will ever taste.

You should be able to simmer unattended all day on low heat if the meat is prethawed, but test this out with your particular crockpot.

Rick and Judy Williams
Viroqua, Wisconsin
www.mistyridgefarm.com

SWEET GRASS FARM'S
THREE–INGREDIENT OVEN DINNER

I tend to use any boneless meat (beef, veal or pork) in bite-sized pieces or ground meat, but chicken or rabbit pieces would work fine, too.

1 pound meat chunks
1 cup brown rice
2 cups medium salsa
Water*

Place all ingredients into roasting pan. Stir briefly to moisten rice and mix ingredients. Cover. Bake 1½ hours at 350 degrees.

 * Use the quantity needed to cook the rice minus the fluid of the salsa. For brown rice, I need 3 cups of fluid, so I use 2 cups salsa and 1 cup water. White rice requires less liquid, so maybe the salsa would do.

Wendy Gornick
Vernon, New York
wgornick@born.com

SKAGIT RIVER RANCH'S
BEEF BRISKET WITH CARAMELIZED ONIONS

1 beef brisket, 4 to 5 pounds
2 teaspoons flour
Lots of coarse pepper
1 tablespoon oil
8 onions, halved and thickly
  sliced
2 heaping tablespoons tomato
  paste
1 heaping teaspoon salt
4 cloves garlic, roughly chopped

Brisket is the muscle between the shoulder and foreleg of the beef. It gets lots of use when it's on the hoof so it needs long slow cooking to make it tender. Most briskets are made into corned beef, but fresh ones are delicious—the ultimate in pot roasts.

I like to cook this recipe the day before because of the mysterious boost in flavor that comes when the meat is cooked with tomato and allowed to rest overnight.
—Eiko Vojkovich

Preheat the oven to 300 degrees. Remove the visible fat from the outside of the brisket. Don't worry about the fat that goes inside. Dry the meat with paper towels and dust with flour.

Heat the oil in a large skillet on medium high. Brown both sides of the roast. Remove the brisket to a baking sheet or other large pan.

Add the onions to the pan on medium-low heat and stir to brown and caramelize. Cook 15 to 20 minutes or until the onions are soft and brown, but not burned. Scrape into a roasting pan and place the browned meat on top. Spread the tomato paste on top of the brisket like frosting. Sprinkle with salt and more pepper. Scatter the garlic on top.

Cover with foil and cook 2 hours. Remove the meat to a cutting board and slice across the grain into ¼–inch slices. This will be a little strange because the grain runs crosswise on a brisket. (That's

why corned beef is so often tough and stringy – it's just cut wrong!)
You may want to cut the whole thing in half across the middle so the
slices won't be long and unwieldy. Re-form the roast in the pan and
cook another 2 hours.

I refrigerate it after slicing. Before serving I add carrots, potatoes,
turnips, etc., and cook it the last 2 hours. The onions make a lovely
thick sauce that's delicious on mashed potatoes spiked with a little
horseradish. Serves 8.

*If you don't want to do all of the above, here is the easier version:
Simply rub these spices (our family's favorite combination) all over
the brisket:*

1 tablespoon sea salt
2 teaspoons paprika
3 teaspoons of crushed garlic
2 teaspoons of black pepper
Pinch of white pepper

Put it on a low heat barbeque at about 200 degrees for 2 hours to
get a good smoke flavor, then bake in the oven at 225 degrees for 8
hours. Slice thin across the grain and serve with your favorite
veggies.

*George and Eiko Vojkovich
Sedro Woolley, Washington
www.skagitriverranch.com*

T.O. CATTLE COMPANY'S
BEEF AND NOODLE CASSEROLE

6 ounces dried egg noodles
4 tablespoons (½ stick) unsalted butter
2 tablespoons unbleached, all-purpose flour
2 cups milk
Salt to taste
Ground white pepper to taste

1 cup finely chopped red or yellow onion
¾ cup finely chopped red or green sweet pepper
1 tablespoon minced or pressed garlic
1½ pounds ground beef
½ pound fresh mushrooms, finely chopped
3 tablespoons top quality chili powder
Freshly ground black pepper
Ground cayenne pepper

2 cups homemade tomato sauce, or one 15–ounce can
   tomato sauce
2 cups homemade creamed corn, or one 17–ounce can
   cream-style corn
1 cup (about 8 ounces) freshly grated cheddar cheese

Preheat oven to 350 degrees.

In large pot, bring 2 quarts water to boil over high heat. Add the noodles and cook until al dente, about 12 minutes. Drain and rinse in cold water to halt cooking and keep the strands separated. Set aside.

To make a white sauce, melt 2 tablespoons of the butter in saucepan over medium-high heat. Add the flour, blend well and cook, stirring until bubbly, about 1 minute. Slowly stir the milk into the flour and butter mixture with a wire whisk. Bring to a boil, reduce heat to medium, and cook, stirring constantly, until thickened, about 5 to 6 minutes. Remove from heat, season to taste with white pepper, and reserve.

Assemble the meat mixture. Heat the remaining 2 tablespoons of butter in a sauté pan or skillet over medium-high heat. Add the onion and sweet pepper and sauté until soft, about 5 minutes. Add the garlic and sauté 1 minute longer. Stir in the ground beef and mushrooms and sauté just until the meat loses its raw meat color, about 5 minutes. Stir in the chili powder. Remove from heat and season to taste with salt, black pepper, and cayenne pepper.

Butter a 2 ½ quart oven-proof casserole dish. Arrange about half of the noodles in the casserole. Cover with half of the meat mixture, half of the tomato sauce, and half of the corn. Add the remaining noodles, meat, tomato sauce, and corn in the same order. Cover the top with the reserved white sauce and sprinkle with the cheeses. Bake until bubbly, about 1 to 1 ½ hours. Serves 6 hungry cowboys.

Joe and Julie Morris
San Juan Bautista, California
www.morrisgrassfed.com

T.O. CATTLE COMPANY'S
SWISS STEAK

This one is from Julie's mom. It's a quick and delicious meal for working parents!

2 pounds beef Swiss steak
2 tablespoons flour
1 teaspoon salt
½ teaspoon each salt, pepper, paprika, and dry mustard, mixed together
¼ cup vegetable oil
3 tablespoons butter
½ cup chopped onion
1 clove garlic, pressed
¾ cup water
3 tablespoons soy sauce
3 tablespoons brown sugar
¾ cup sour cream
1 bag stroganoff noodles

Preheat oven to 300 degrees. Cut meat into serving size pieces. Dust with flour and pound with meat mallet. Sprinkle with paprika mixture. Heat oil in large, deep skillet. Add butter. Sear steak on one side. Add onion, garlic, water, soy sauce, brown sugar, and sour cream. Stir to blend. Cover and bake 30 to 45 minutes until tender. Serve over cooked noodles. Serves 6.

Joe and Julie Morris
San Juan Bautista, California
www.morrisgrassfed.com

T.O. CATTLE COMPANY'S
BAKED STEAK

This recipe comes from Joe's mom. It's an easy one, great for entertaining because you have time to enjoy your company.

Chuck roast or London broil, cut thick, about 2 inches
Onions
Tomatoes
A bit of garlic
Worcestershire sauce
Dry or Dijon mustard
Salt and pepper to taste

Salt and pepper meat and broil 10 minutes on each side. Sauté onions, mushrooms, and garlic while meat is broiling. Remove roast, dribble Worcestershire and mustard on top. Put sliced tomatoes and sautéed onions, garlic, and mushrooms on top of meat.

Bake in oven for a half hour at 350 degrees. Serve warm, with a fresh green salad, garlic bread, and glass of red Chianti.

Joe and Julie Morris
San Juan Bautista, California
www.morrisgrassfed.com

OAK MOON FARM
LAB NUE (THAI GROUND BEEF SALAD)

Jack first came across this recipe when he was a Peace Corps Volunteer in Thailand. It makes a great summertime salad, or a potluck "dish to pass." Fish sauce, Thai Jasmine Rice, ganglal powder and toasted rice powder can be found in any Asian food market, or in the Asian section of larger supermarkets.

1 pound ground beef
¼ cup fish sauce
½ cup lime juice
1 tablespoon ganglal powder (found in Asian stores)
2 tablespoons toasted rice powder
1 teaspoon red pepper flakes
1 bunch green onions, white and green parts, cut diagonally into ⅛-inch pieces
½ cup mint leaves
10 cabbage leaves, cut into thirds
Thai Jasmine rice

Cook the rice according to the directions on the package.

Heat a skillet or wok and fry the ground beef until the red color disappears. Set aside in a non-reactive bowl and allow to cool. Stir the fish sauce and lime juice into the ground beef. Add the ganglal powder, toasted rice powder, and red pepper and stir. Toss the green onions and mint leaves into the ground beef mixture.

To eat, scoop up a small portion of the beef mixture with a cut cabbage leaf. Serve with cooked Thai Jasmine rice.

Jack and Martha Knorek
Olivet, Michigan
www.oakmoonfarm.com

RIVER RUN FARM'S
FETA & HERB STUFFED BURGERS

1 pound ground beef from grass-fed beef
1 cup chopped spinach
$^1/_3$ cup chopped or crumbled feta cheese
1 heaping tablespoon fresh oregano, coarsely chopped
Salt and pepper

Mix feta, oregano, and spinach in a small bowl and set aside.

Divide ground beef into three equal parts. Form into ball shapes, then press flat. Place $^1/_3$ of the feta mixture in the middle of each patty, and form into a ball again around the mixture. Press into firm patties again, making sure not to let stuffing show by redistributing ground beef as necessary to make it as even as possible. Sprinkle with salt and pepper and grill as normal.

Serving suggestions: serve with a fresh herb salad and roasted new potatoes. Or serve on an onion bun with creative condiments such as alfalfa sprouts, tomatoes, sliced cucumbers, spinach leaves. Serves 3.

James and Ellen Girt
Clatskanie, Oregon
info@riverrunfarm.com
www.riverrunfarm.com

KAREN'S GRASSLAND MEATS'
ARIZONA SUR SHREDDED BEEF

This basic recipe is easily adjusted to make barbecue beef or green chile beef by varying the seasonings. It freezes fabulously. I use ½ pound of meat per person—people can't stop eating this!

Chuck roast
Fresh garlic
Cumin
Red chile powder or paste

Use either a slow cooker/roaster, or a roasting pan with a tight fitting lid. Cut the chuck roast as necessary to fit the pan.

Sprinkle the roast with cumin and red chili (or add chile paste) and add fresh garlic cloves, cut in half, to taste. Vary the amount of chile for mild to hot, or omit it altogether. We are very influenced by Mexican cooking and probably like hotter seasoning than our northern neighbors, so we suggest you add chile according to your taste. Add salt and pepper after cooking—you'll be surprised at how little you'll need. Add about an inch of water to the pan. Use a tight-fitting lid.

In a slow cooker, cook on high for at least 12 hours. If you are using a roasting pan, cook at 300 degrees for about 8 hours or until beef shreds with a fork. As soon as the meat is removed from the oven or the slow cooker is turned off, take two forks and shred the beef immediately in the pan it was cooked in. As you pull the meat apart with the forks, it will absorb any liquid in the pan. This can be served immediately with warm corn or flour tortillas, over beans on a tostada, in tacos or enchiladas, or in a taco salad.

Karen and Clay Riggs
Willcox, Arizona
cimarron@vtc.net

OSWALD CATTLE COMPANY'S
STIR-FRIED BEEF AND BROCCOLI

This is a recipe we give to new customers. It's one of our favorites and a great way to hook those who are new to grass-fed beef.

1½ pounds round steak cut crosswise in thin slices
½ to ¾ cups water, divided
½ cup soy sauce
2 tablespoons packed brown sugar
3 tablespoons cooking sherry, wine or wine vinegar
2 cloves garlic, crushed
1 teaspoon ginger
1 teaspoon cornstarch
1 bunch of broccoli (about 4 cups)
1 large onion
3 tablespoons oil

Combine soy sauce, sugar, sherry, garlic, ginger, cornstarch, and one-half of the water and pour over sliced steak. Let marinate for at least 10 minutes. Drain, reserving the marinade.

Brown the steak slices in a skillet. Remove the browned meat from the pan and set aside. Brown the broccoli and onion lightly. Add remaining water and steam until broccoli is crisp and tender. Return the meat to skillet with remaining marinade and simmer. Serve over rice.

Steve and Nancy Oswald
Cotopaxi, Colorado
steveo@bwn.net

T.O. CATTLE COMPANY'S
SUMMER BEEF SALAD WITH ARUGULA & RED ONIONS

2 teaspoons Dijon mustard
2 teaspoons Balsamic vinegar
1 teaspoon lemon juice
¼ teaspoon sea salt
¼ teaspoon freshly ground black pepper
¼ cup olive oil
2 tablespoons fresh cilantro, chopped
½ red onion, sliced
¼ pound green beans, halved
½ pound arugula, washed
1 cup bean sprouts
1 beef skirt or flank steak, barbecued and sliced

In a large bowl, whisk the mustard, vinegar, lemon juice, salt, pepper, oil, and cilantro. Add the onion, green beans, arugula, and bean sprouts and toss well. Divide among four plates and top with beef slices. Serves 4.

Joe and Julie Morris
San Juan Bautista, California
www.morrisgrassfed.com

OAK MOON FARM'S
SLOPPY JOES

It took a lot of experimenting, but I finally arrived at a Sloppy Joe recipe that the entire family likes!

2 pounds ground beef
1 small onion, chopped
  (optional)
1¼ cups water
2 beef bouillon cubes
½ cup ketchup
2 tablespoons spicy brown
  mustard
3 tablespoons cider vinegar
1 tablespoon Worcestershire
  sauce
3 tablespoons orange juice
3 tablespoons brown sugar,
  packed
2 tablespoons paprika
1 teaspoon black pepper
1 tablespoon sweet pickle relish (optional)

I have noticed that my customers are initially shocked at the amount of ground beef that comes with a side or a quarter of beef — and dismayed that the carcass is not mostly T-bone steaks!

I now educate my customers before the sale to avoid any surprises; I also provide some recipes. It takes a creative cook to utilize that much ground beef, which is typically 30 to 35% of what actually gets delivered. —Jack Knorek

Brown the ground beef; add the chopped onion if you are using it. Add the water and bouillon cubes. Simmer until the bouillon cubes are dissolved. Add the remaining ingredients and simmer until the desired consistency is achieved. Serve on hamburger buns.

Jack and Martha Knorek
Olivet, Michigan
www.oakmoonfarm.com

SWEET GRASS FARM'S
SUPER SLOPPY JOES

1 pound lean ground beef, pork, lamb, veal, or turkey
½ cup chopped onion
1 tablespoon prepared mustard
2 to 3 teaspoons chili powder
1 8–ounce can tomato sauce
1 6–ounce can tomato juice
½ cup shredded carrot
⅓ cup bulgur wheat
6 whole wheat hamburger buns, split and toasted
4 ounces (½ cup) shredded cheddar cheese

Cook the meat and onion in a 10–inch skillet until the meat is brown and the onion is tender. Drain off any excess fat. Stir in the mustard and chili powder. Cook and stir for 1 minute.

Add tomato sauce, juice, carrot, and wheat. Bring mixture to boiling; reduce heat. Simmer mixture, uncovered, for 10 minutes, stirring occasionally. Meanwhile, toast buns.

To serve, spoon the meat mixture over the buns and sprinkle each sandwich with shredded cheese. Serves 6.

Wendy Gornick
Vernon, New York
wgornick@born.com

SWEET GRASS FARM'S
TENDER BEEF HEART WITH GRAVY

1½ pounds beef heart, trimmed of fat
1 cup buttermilk
2 large onions, chopped
4 cloves of garlic, minced
3 tablespoons oil
10-ounce can of mushroom, onion, or beef gravy
¼ teaspoon powdered ginger
Salt and pepper to taste

Place the meat in a flat baking dish, then cover it a bit more than halfway with the buttermilk. Soak in a cool place for at least 1 hour, turning every ½ hour or so. It will hold overnight in the refrigerator.

About 1½ hours before serving, sauté the onions and garlic in the oil in a large skillet over medium heat while you cut the meat into uniform ¼-inch dice. Add the meat to the skillet and toss to blend. Stir in the gravy, cover the pan, and turn heat to low. Simmer, stirring frequently, for about 45 to 50 minutes, or until the meat is tender.

Gravy will thin down after cooking awhile, then thicken again; you may want to add a splash of water if it gets too thick. Stir in ginger, then taste for salt and pepper.

Delicious served with hot whipped potatoes. Serves 6.

Wendy Gornick
Vernon, New York
wgornick@born.com

BISON & VENISON RECIPES

SMOKY HILL BISON COMPANY'S
BAKED BISON STEW

14 ½ ounce can diced tomatoes, undrained
(*I suggest Del Monte Zesty Tomato)*
1 cup water
3 tablespoons quick-cooking tapioca
2 teaspoons sugar
1 ½ teaspoons salt
½ teaspoon pepper
2 pounds bison stew meat
4 medium carrots cut into 1–inch chunks
3 medium potatoes, peeled and quartered
2 celery ribs cut into $^3/_4$ –inch chunks
1 medium onion, cut into chunks
1 slice bread, cubed

Why eat bison? Because it's tender, tasty and healthy!

From a steak to a burger, this excellent source of protein is low in fat, and has as much potassium as a banana, and as much calcium as a glass of milk.

This clean sweet meat is easy to cook by itself, or used in your favorite recipes.   —Linda Hubalek

In a large bowl, combine the first six ingredients. Add remaining ingredients, mix well, and pour into a greased 13 x 9 inch pan or 3-quart baking dish. Cover and bake at 325 degrees for 2 ½ to 3 hours, or until meat and vegetables are tender. Serve in bowls. Serves 6 to 8.

Verne and Linda Hubalek
Lindsborg, Kansas
www.bisonfarm.com

SMOKY HILL BISON COMPANY'S
BISON MEAT LOAF

½ cup chopped onion
1 tablespoon butter or margarine
2 eggs, beaten
1 cup milk
¾ cup quick-cooking or rolled oats
1 tablespoon chopped fresh parsley
2 teaspoons salt
½ teaspoon dried savory or favorite herb
¼ teaspoon pepper
2 to 2 ½ pounds bison ground burger

Glaze:
½ cup ketchup
2 tablespoons brown sugar
½ teaspoon Worcestershire sauce
1 teaspoon yellow mustard

In a small skillet, sauté onion in butter until transparent. In a large bowl, combine onion with eggs, milk, oats, parsley, and seasonings. Add ground bison and mix well. Press into an 8 ½ x 4 ½ inch loaf pan lined with waxed paper. Refrigerate for 2 hours.

Unmold loaf into a shallow baking pan. Bake at 325 degrees for 30 minutes. Meanwhile, combine glaze ingredients. Remove loaf from oven. Brush on the glaze and return to oven. Bake 1 hour or until done. Serves 10 to 12.

Verne and Linda Hubalek
Lindsborg, Kansas
www.bisonfarm.com

BUFFALO GROVES'
TRI TIP ROAST

A great meal we enjoy with rice and a cool fruit salad.

Tri Tip buffalo roast
1 small can mandarin oranges
2 tablespoons teriyaki sauce
¼ cup honey

Start with a Tri Tip roast. Trim away connective tissue or silver skin. Blend together oranges, teriyaki sauce and honey together lightly in a blender. Marinate the roast for 1 hour (or more) in this mixture.

> Our commitment at Buffalo Groves is to work together as a family, raising our bison in the truest harmony with nature. We manage our land and our herds responsibly.
>
> We welcome visitors. We want to show you how our work provides this wonderfully healthy meat!
>
> —David and Marlene

Heat your barbecue to medium and put the Tri Tip on the top rack. Baste and turn the roast about every 10 minutes. Depending on the size of the roast and your barbecue, it may cook from 1½ – 2½ hours (average 2 hours). Check it with a meat thermometer and remove it at no more than 140 degrees, then let it sit for 5 to 10 minutes before slicing.

David and Marlene Groves
Kiowa, Colorado
www.buffalogroves.com

BUFFALO GROVES'
EASY BAKED BUFFALO ENCHILADAS

This is a great meal for gatherings, we like to serve it with beans and rice.

2 pounds of ground buffalo
½ to 1 diced onion
2 small cans of diced green chilies.
28–ounce can red enchilada sauce
12 to 16 corn tortillas, each cut into 6 triangle wedges
2 to 3 cups of grated cheddar cheese
½ to 1 cup of sliced black olives

Cook the buffalo and onion together in a non-stick or lightly greased skillet. After the meat is cooked, add diced green chilies.

Spray a rectangular baking pan with non-stick spray, then spread ½ cup of the enchilada sauce over the pan bottom and layer about half of the tortilla wedges in the pan. Spoon on the meat mixture, then layer the remaining tortillas. Level the layers with a big spoon or spatula (or your hands), then add all but ½ cup of the enchilada sauce. It may look like a lot of sauce, but cover it with foil and let the pan sit for 60 minutes; the tortillas will absorb some of the sauce. Put the pan in a preheated 350 oven and bake it for 60 minutes.

Remove the foil, add the rest of the sauce, and 2 to 3 cups of grated cheddar cheese. Top it with sliced black olives. Pop the whole works back in the oven to melt the cheese.

David and Marlene Groves
Kiowa, Colorado
www.buffalogroves.com

FALLOW HOLLOW DEER FARM'S
VENISON FAJITAS

2 pounds venison roast
3 tablespoons vegetable oil
¼ cup cider vinegar
1 teaspoon sugar
1 teaspoon dried oregano
1 teaspoon chili powder
½ teaspoon garlic powder
½ teaspoon salt
¼ teaspoon black pepper
Dash of red pepper
2 large onions
2 large bell peppers (red or green)
12 large soft tortilla shells

Slice venison into very thin strips. Slice onions and cut peppers into strips. Heat oil in a large stir-fry type pan over medium-high heat. Add venison and quickly brown. Add onions and peppers and fry until crisp cooked. Reduce heat to low. Add vinegar, sugar, oregano, chili powder, garlic, salt, and peppers. Simmer until vegetables have reached desired tenderness.

Serve beef mixture in center of warmed tortilla shells. Optional toppings include salsa or picante sauce, sour cream, grated cheeses, and guacamole.

Martha Goodsell
Candor, New York
info@fallowhollow.com
www.fallowhollow.com

FALLOW HOLLOW DEER FARM'S
HUNTER STYLE CHILI

Venison really holds spices used in cooking. I love it for Mexican style cooking and so do our four kids—especially venison fajitas and tacos. Here's a chili recipe I've worked on over the years. Most folks say it's the best they've ever had. You be the judge!

3 pounds ground venison
1 tablespoon vegetable oil
3 large onions
3 large green peppers
1 ½ cups shredded carrot
3 cloves garlic, crushed
3 tablespoons chili powder
3 teaspoons beef bouillon
3 teaspoons ground cumin
3 teaspoons dried oregano
½ teaspoon red cayenne pepper
1 teaspoon hot sauce
2 28–ounce cans tomato sauce
1 28–ounce can kidney beans

Brown venison in heavy skillet. Remove browned venison to crockpot. In same heavy skillet add oil, peppers, onion, carrots and garlic. Cook until tender and vegetables begin to brown. Add vegetables to venison in crockpot. Add all remaining ingredients to crockpot and stir. Cover and simmer 4 hours over low heat.

Martha Goodsell
Candor, New York
info@fallowhollow.com
www.fallowhollow.com

FALLOW HOLLOW DEER FARM'S
SPINACH–FETA VENISON SPIRALS

All those cuts not considered prime don't have to end up in ground, stews, or sausages. Here's a filled roast from the neck.

1 ½ pounds venison neck roast
1 teaspoon salt
½ teaspoon pepper
¼ teaspoon garlic powder
½ teaspoon basil
½ teaspoon chopped parsley
½ cup water
½ cup white wine
1 cup steamed spinach
¹/₃ cup crumbled feta cheese

To cut this, start at the middle of the lower side of the neck and cut the meat off the bone going up and around. You'll end up with a flat piece 14 by 8 inches, depending upon the size of your deer. Flatten neck to uniform thickness. Season with salt and pepper. In a small bowl combine spinach, cheese, garlic, parsley, and basil. Spread lengthwise onto half the roast. Roll roast beginning at the filling end. (There should be no filling in the outermost roll.) Secure with butcher's twine.

In a Dutch oven, brown the rolled venison on all sides, then remove roast. Add water and wine to deglaze pan. Add roast, cover, and bake 1½ hours at 325 degrees. Remove from pan and let rest before slicing.

Martha Goodsell
Candor, New York
info@fallowhollow.com

LAMB & VEAL RECIPES

THE ROCK GARDEN'S
LAMB WITH WINE AND MOREL GRAVY

The morels are what give this dish its unique, rich flavor. In a pinch, shiitake mushrooms can be substituted for all or part of the morels.

1 lamb shoulder or leg roast, well trimmed

1 cup sweet red or rosé wine (We use a homecrafted apple and
   plum wine but any sweet commercial wine will do.)

2 cups water

½ cup dried morel mushrooms (Use ¼ cup if using fresh morels or
   other mushrooms.)

2 tablespoons dried minced garlic

2 teaspoons cornstarch

Pour wine and water over roast. Add morel mushrooms and dried minced garlic. (To substitute fresh garlic, use one whole head peeled and crushed.) Bake at 325 degrees, allowing 30 minutes for each pound of lamb.

Lift roast from pan and quickly blend cornstarch mixed with 2 teaspoons water into hot drippings to thicken. Add salt to taste.

Skip and Christy Hensler
Newport, Washington
www.povn.com/rock/

SWEET GRASS FARM'S
WINTER LAMB STEW

This stew will freeze well for about 2 months.

½ cup diced slab bacon (about 4 ounces)
3 pounds boneless lamb, cut into 1–inch cubes
¼ cup flour
1 tablespoon sugar
1 teaspoon salt
¼ teaspoon pepper
¼ cup chopped shallots or green onions
2 cloves garlic, minced
1 28–ounce can whole tomatoes
2½ cups condensed beef broth or lamb broth made from bones
1 teaspoon leaf rosemary, crumbled
½ teaspoon leaf thyme, crumbled
2 tablespoons butter
12 pearl onions (about ¾ pound)
4 medium turnips (about 1 pound), pared and quartered
3 medium sweet potatoes (about 1 pound), pared, halved
   lengthwise, then cut into 1–inch slices
4 large carrots, halved and cut into 2-inch pieces
1 10–ounce package frozen peas

Cook bacon slowly in a 4–quart saucepan until fat is rendered and pieces are brown. Remove with slotted spoon to paper toweling; drain.

Combine lamb cubes with flour, sugar, salt and pepper in a large bowl; toss to coat. Brown lamb, a few pieces at a time, in bacon drippings. Remove pieces as they brown to a Dutch oven.

Pour off all but 1 tablespoon of the drippings from the saucepan then add shallots and garlic. Sauté, stirring often, until tender, about 2 minutes. Stir in tomatoes, broth, rosemary, and thyme. Bring to boiling, stirring constantly to loosen browned bits in the saucepan. Add to lamb along with bacon. Cover. Bake in a moderate 350–degree oven for 1 hour.

While lamb bakes, heat butter in the same saucepan; add onions, turnips and sweet potatoes. Sauté, stirring 10 minutes or until vegetables are lightly browned and glazed.

Add glazed vegetables and carrots to lamb, pushing them down under liquid; cover. Bake an additional 30 minutes or until lamb is tender and vegetables are soft but not mushy. Stir in peas. Serves 8.

Wendy Gornick
Vernon, New York
wgornick@born.com

3-CORNER FIELD FARM'S
TAJINE D'AGNEAU AU POIRES ET AU MIEL - BRAISED LAMB SHOULDER WITH PEARS & HONEY

We got this "well-traveled" recipe from my French teacher and friend, Odile Grand-Clement. She got the recipe from a friend in North Africa. Tajine is a particular type of Moroccan stew. We have fondly shared this recipe with hundreds of customers in New York City who buy our grassfed lamb at the green market. They, in turn, have shared it with their friends everywhere.

2 to 3 pounds boneless lamb shoulder
2 pounds fresh pears
4 medium onions
4 tablespoons butter
5 tablespoons honey
1 tablespoon cinnamon
1 pinch saffron
Salt and fresh ground pepper

Cut the lamb into cubes about 1–inch square. Melt the butter in a Dutch oven or covered casserole, then add lamb, salt, pepper, cinnamon, and saffron. Mix well and sauté lamb until brown. Cover meat with water. Cook covered for 30 minutes.

Peel the onions. Cut into large pieces. Add to the lamb mixture. Cover and cook an additional 30 minutes.

When the lamb is thoroughly cooked and tender, perhaps an additional 15 to 30 minutes, remove the lamb (only) from the casserole. Peel the pears. Cut into large pieces. Add pears to the casserole along with the honey. Cook over medium heat for about 20 minutes until the pears are just becoming tender.

Add the lamb back to the casserole and cook for another 10 minutes to blend all the flavors. At this point, if the sauce is too thin, it can be reduced by temporarily removing it from the meat, pears, and onion mixture and cooking it in a separate saucepan until it thickens. Then add the thickened sauce back to the lamb, pears and onions. Serve with couscous. Serves 6.

When we first bought our property it was our dream to run it one day as a full-time farm. We had the opportunity to live in France and pretty much closed down our farm for the three years we were away. While living in France we became more knowledge-able about good quality meat and cheeses and were inspired to start our sheep dairy when we returned.

Karen Weinberg and Paul Borghard
Shushan, New York
www.dairysheepfarm.com

THIRTEEN MILE FARM'S
LAMB DOGS (OR LOAF)

1 pound ground lamb

1 egg

½ cup cooked quinoa (You can substitute cooked rice or raw rolled oats, but quinoa is best.)

¼ cup grated parmesan cheese (grated grass-fed sheep cheese if you can get it!)

¼ cup coarsely ground corn meal

⅓ cup spiced tomato sauce

⅓ cup chopped fresh parsley

⅓ cup chopped fresh mint

1 tablespoon lemon pepper

1 tablespoon chopped fresh rosemary

1 tablespoon chopped fresh oregano

Mix all of the ingredients together, then shape into 10 small elongated dogs. Grill or roast the dogs in the oven, or shape into two small loaves and set on cast iron skillet or other heavy-weight pan sprinkled with coarse corn meal. Cover with a glaze made from the following:

½ cup spiced tomato sauce

1 tablespoon mustard

¼ cup brown sugar

¼ cup grated parmesan cheese

Brush glaze onto loaves, and roast in a 375–degree oven for about 1 hour. Roast hotter and faster for a good crust on the outside.

Becky Weed and David Tyler
Belgrade, Montana
www.lambandwool.com

WINDSWEPT FARM'S
LAMBURGERS!

Lamburgers can be broiled, but grilling is far better. I prefer them medium rare. Please don't overcook – it will make them too dry. I prefer crusty French rolls but if you only have regular buns, try toasting them. Dijon mustard, tomato and onion makes for great eating. Enjoy!

1 pound lean ground lamb
1 teaspoon dry or 1 tablespoon fresh, finely chopped mint (I prefer peppermint)
½ teaspoon dry or 2 teaspoons fresh, finely chopped oregano
½ teaspoon salt, or to taste

Mix all ingredients together and let stand for at least 30 minutes to blend flavors. Shape into two or three patties and grill.

We have a flock of sixty Katahdin ewes. They have delicious, mild, exceptionally tender meat despite the fact that they get no grain whatsoever. They finish extremely well on grass, even in years where the summers are quite dry.

If everyone who ever tried lamb, could have grass fed Katahdin meat, the lamb market would be zooming along!

—Jeanne Weaver

Jeanne Weaver
Williamston, Michigan
weaver3@shiatel.tds.net
www.windsweptfarms.com/

SWEET GRASS FARM'S
POACHED VEAL TONGUE

This method also works for beef or pork tongues.

1 calf's tongue, about 1¼ pounds
4 cups water, or enough to cover
¼ cup coarsely chopped celery
½ cup coarsely chopped onion
½ cup carrot cut into rounds
1 bay leaf
2 sprigs fresh thyme or ½ teaspoon dried
4 sprigs fresh parsley
1 whole clove
Salt to taste
12 crushed peppercorns
1 clove garlic, peeled

Place the tongue in a kettle and add cold water to cover. Bring to a boil and simmer about 5 minutes. Drain.

Return the tongue to a clean kettle. Add the 4 cups water and all the remaining ingredients. Bring to the boil and simmer until quite tender throughout, about 1½ hours.

Let the tongue cool in its liquid till lukewarm. Serve lukewarm or cold. To serve, cut the tongue into ¼–inch slices and serve with a bit of chutney or salsa. Serves 2 as a main dish or 4 as an appetizer.

Wendy Gornick
Vernon, New York
wgornick@born.com

SWEET GRASS FARM'S
CITRUS-RUBBED VEAL CHOPS
WITH SUNSHINE SALSA

You can also make a good salsa using lemon peel, lemon juice and orange segments instead of the lime and mango.

6 veal loin or rib chops, well-trimmed and cut 1–inch thick
  (about 8 ounces each)
½ teaspoon salt
½ teaspoon grated lime peel

Salsa:
1 mango, peeled, seeded, and cut into ½–inch pieces
½ cup prepared salsa
¼ cup minced red onion
2 tablespoons fresh lime juice

Combine salsa ingredients in a saucepan and bring to a medium boil. Cover and refrigerate. Serve chops with salsa.

Total preparation and cooking time is 25 minutes.

Wendy Gornick
Vernon, New York
wgornick@born.com

SAP BUSH HOLLOW FARM'S
SHOULDER CHOPS WITH CARDAMOM, APPLES, AND APRICOTS

Here's an elegant little way to prepare tasty shoulder chops. The recipe serves two, but can easily be doubled or tripled.

2 lamb shoulder chops or leg chops

½ teaspoon ground cardamom
½ teaspoon ground cinnamon
½ teaspoon cayenne pepper
¼ teaspoon ground cloves
1 teaspoon salt

2 tablespoons olive oil
2 onions, cut into ¼–inch wedges
1 teaspoon ground ginger
1 cup water
1 apple, peeled and sliced
$^2/_3$ cup dried apricots
4 teaspoons honey

Thoroughly combine the cardamom, cinnamon, cayenne pepper, cloves and salt in a small bowl. Rub the mixture into both sides of the lamb chops. Heat the olive oil in a large pot over a medium flame. Sear the chops 2 to 3 minutes per side, then remove. Add the onions and sauté until translucent. Add the apricots, ginger, apples and water.

Cook over medium heat, stirring constantly for one minute, then set the chops on top of the onions and fruit. Cover and simmer over low heat for two hours, until the chops are fork tender. Turn the heat off and allow the chops to rest for 5 minutes. Place the chops on plates, top with the onion and fruit mixture, then drizzle each chop with 2 teaspoons of honey. Serves 2.

Crock pot variation: After searing the chops, stir together the onions, ginger, water (reduce the amount to ½ cup), apple, and apricots in a crock pot. Place the browned chops on top, and cook on low for 6 hours, or until the meat pulls easily from the bone.

As this book was going to press, we learned that Shannon Hayes has written a book about cooking pasture-raised meat that will be published in the fall of 2004. The book contains recipes, profiles of grassfarmers, and contact information for pastured-meat farmers around the country. It also explains appropriate cooking techniques and information about how to choose and purchase meat from a pasture-based farm.Learn more about the book on Shannon's website: www.shannonhayes.info

Shannon Hayes
Warnerville, New York
shayes@midtel.net

SAP BUSH HOLLOW FARM'S
ROASTED LEG OF LAMB OR LOIN ROAST

Herb Paste:

2 cloves garlic

1 tablespoon coarse salt

2 teaspoons fresh ground
  pepper

1 tablespoon dried rosemary

2 teaspoons dried thyme

½ teaspoon dried mustard

6 tablespoons olive oil

5 to 6 pound leg of lamb, or a
  2 pound loin roast

The leg of lamb is a magnificent feast, suitable for the most appreciative dinner companions.

Unfortunately, many people have a tendency to overcook it, when it is really best served rosy and rare. So if you like nice juicy lamb, be sure to use your meat thermometer.

The loin roast is a significantly more expensive roast, but it is very tender and extremely elegant. —Shannon Hayes

Combine the herb paste ingredients in a food processor and puree. (If you don't have a food processor, just mince the garlic as finely as possible and stir it in with the other ingredients.) Rub all over the leg, and allow it to rest at room temperature for an hour or two, or overnight (covered with plastic wrap) in the refrigerator.

Preheat the oven to 500 degrees. Place the leg of lamb in a large roasting pan in the oven, then immediately reduce the heat to 250 degrees. Continue roasting to 120 degrees for a rare roast, 130 for medium, or 140 for well-done. Cooking times vary, but allow at least two and a half hours at 250 degrees for a medium–rare 5 ½ pound leg. Remove the lamb from the oven, cover loosely with foil, and let it rest for at least 15 minutes before serving. The lamb will continue to cook during this time, and the temperature will rise another 5 to 10 degrees.

Shannon Hayes
Warnerville, New York
shayes@midtel.net

PORK RECIPES

GENESIS FARMING'S
VERMONT PORK ROAST WITH SAUERKRAUT

Pork Roast
1 to 1½ quarts naturally fermented raw sauerkraut
Lard

Preheat oven to 325 degrees. Brown the roast on all sides on medium high heat in a roasting pan, using some lard if necessary. Set about a cup of sauerkraut aside in the refrigerator and use the remainder to surround the roast.

Cover and place in oven. Cook until tender, about 2 to 4 hours, depending on size. Check every ½ hour for tenderness and add water if liquid is low.

Delicious with hot mashed or baked potatoes topped with butter from grassfed cows and the cold sauerkraut.

We raise our pigs in portable pens on grass and move them to fresh pasture daily. In addition to organic grain, we are fortunate to have fresh salt-free whey from a national award winning cheese maker located nearby. This combination results in darker colored pork, richer in flavor and firmer in texture than what you may be used to seeing.

Richard and Vicky Lynn Palmer
Corinth, Vermont
palmers@genesisfarming.com

SAP BUSH HOLLOW FARM'S
HONEY GLAZED RIB ROAST
WITH APPLE WALNUT STUFFING

Pork rib roasts really lend themselves well to flashy cooking, so here's a fun recipe to dazzle your dinner guests!

1 4–bone pork rib roast
1 tablespoon coarse salt
2 teaspoons ground black pepper
1 tablespoon rubbed sage

For the stuffing:
2 tablespoons butter
1 small onion, minced
1 small apple, peeled and finely diced
½ cup raisins
¼ cup dry white wine
¼ cup chopped walnuts
1 teaspoon rubbed sage

½ cup honey
¼ cup lemon juice
¼ cup olive oil

2 tablespoons butter
1 ½ cups chicken broth

Combine coarse salt, black pepper, and sage and rub it into the pork roast. Cover and refrigerate over night.

For the stuffing, melt the butter in a skillet over medium heat. Add the onion and sauté 1 minute. Add the apple and raisins and cook a few minutes longer, until the onions are translucent. Add the wine and simmer until most of the liquid is absorbed. Stir in the sage and walnuts and set aside to cool.

Preheat the oven to 450 degrees. Using a long sharp knife (a fillet knife works well), carve a ¾-inch wide hole through the meatiest part of the roast. Take all of the carved-out meat, dice it, and refrigerate it. Firmly pack the apple walnut stuffing into the hole, making sure it comes through to the other side of the roast. Set the meat in a roasting pan, reserving any extra stuffing.

Whisk together the honey, lemon juice, and olive oil and brush it on the pork. Put the roast in the oven and immediately lower the heat to 300 degrees. Cook, basting 2 or 3 times with the pan juices, for about 2 hours and 45 minutes, or until an instant-read thermometer inserted into the thickest part of the meat (not the stuffing) registers 150 degrees. Thirty minutes before the meat is done, put the extra stuffing in a small, oven-proof dish, cover it with foil, and put it in the oven to bake. Once the internal temperature of the meat is 150 degrees, transfer the roast to a cutting board and tent it loosely with foil.

Set the roasting pan over 2 burners on the stove and turn the heat on medium. Add the 2 tablespoons butter, then the reserved diced pork. Sauté 2 minutes, or until the meat is cooked through. Add the chicken broth, thoroughly blend it with the pan drippings, then simmer until the liquid is reduced to 1 cup, scraping up any browned bits. Carve the pork by cutting between the ribs to make chops. Spoon the pan sauce on top, sprinkle with the extra stuffing, and serve. Serves 4

Shannon Hayes
Warnerville, New York
shayes@midtel.net

GENESIS FARMING'S
PORK BARBECUE

6 to 8 pounds of pork shoulder, cooked and shredded
¾ cup of lard
2 cups cider vinegar
1 tablespoon dry mustard
½ cup onions, chopped
½ cup Worcestershire sauce
2 tablespoons lemon juice
2 tablespoons Tabasco Sauce (or to taste)
1 cup tomato paste
½ teaspoon coarsely ground black pepper
3 to 5 cloves garlic, minced
½ teaspoon honey
2 cups water

Brown the roast on all sides on medium high heat in a roasting pan, using some lard if necessary. Cover and place in oven until tender, approximately 2 to 4 hours, depending on size. Check every ½ hour for tenderness and add water if liquid is low. Remove from oven when meat shreds easily with a fork. Leave in pan or place on cutting board to shred.

Combine remaining ingredients in a 1–quart bowl. Mix well. Add to the meat and simmer on low heat for several hours. Serve on soft sourdough buns like a sandwich. Serves 10

Richard and Vicky Lynn Palmer
Corinth, Vermont
palmers@genesisfarming.com

SWEET GRASS FARM'S
GINGER MAPLE RIBS

2 racks back ribs (about 1½ pounds)
½ cup pure maple syrup
2 tablespoons soy sauce
¼ cup dry sherry
2 garlic cloves, crushed
1 to 2 tablespoons ginger root, peeled and finely minced
2 tablespoons vegetable oil

Place ribs in large saucepan. Cover with water and bring to a boil. Reduce heat and simmer, covered, until fork-tender, about 30 minutes. Refrigerate if not using right away.

For easy grilling, leave rack of ribs in one piece. Meanwhile, prepare marinade by stirring remaining ingredients together in a medium saucepan. Bring to a boil over medium heat and, stirring often, boil gently for 5 minutes to develop flavors. Drain cooked ribs well.

Preheat barbeque and lightly grease grill. Brush ribs with marinade. Place ribs on grill about 6 inches from hot coals. Grill, turning ribs every 5 minutes and basting with remaining marinade, until heated through, about 15 to 20 minutes. Cut into serving size pieces. Serves 6.

Wendy Gornick
Vernon, New York
wgornick@borg.com

WOODBRIDGE FARM'S
HAM STEAK AND EGGS

I am crying just thinking about it...

1 ham steak
Pastured eggs, prepared any style
Butter (cultured butter even better)

Brown the ham steak on each side. When just browned and warm, remove and serve next to eggs. Top the ham steak with some cultured butter.

Steven Bibula
Salem, Connecticut
woodbridgefarm@joimail.com

WOODBRIDGE FARM'S
PORK EGGROLLS

A guest-friendly party food that will command attention. Ratios and ingredients can be freely modified to taste and any unused mixture can be frozen for future use!

1 pound ground pork, unseasoned
1 package eggroll wrappers (twenty wrappers)
1 cup shredded carrots
2 cups shredded green cabbage, any kind
½ cup chopped green onions or leeks
3 scrambled eggs, well cooked and in small pieces
Approximately 4 tablespoons soy sauce
A sprinkle of sesame seeds
Any suitable frying fat

Combine all ingredients. Use your hands for best and fastest results. Fill the wrappers according to package instructions, then flatten them slightly for pan frying (as you would pirogies) until golden brown on each side. Or roll them cylindrically and deep fry for that classic eggroll experience. Serve pretty soon.

Steven Bibula
Salem, Connecticut
woodbridgefarm@joimail.com

SAP BUSH HOLLOW FARM'S
BOSTON BAKED BEANS WITH HAM HOCKS

There is no way around it—baked beans, done well, are an all-day and overnight project. It is possible that they can be done faster in a pressure-cooker, but I am loathe to trust anything that promises to cook food at a speed faster than food naturally cooks. Baked beans are an all-day treat for the senses. They fill your home with warmth from the time you start them on the top of the stove, until the time you pull them from the oven at supper and serve them to your family.

Always be sure to soak your beans overnight before you begin cooking them. If you are concerned about neutralizing the phytic acid in the navy beans, then add 2 tablespoons of yogurt or whey to the soaking water so that the bacteria can break it down while the beans soak. The secret to superlative baked beans lies in using plenty of ham hocks. They impart incredible flavor, and make for heartier fare.

1 pound navy beans, soaked over night
2 tablespoons yogurt or whey (optional)
3 quarts water
1 medium onion, cut into wedges
½ cup molasses
2 tablespoons brown sugar
½ teaspoon mustard
¼ teaspoon ginger
¼ teaspoon allspice
2 to 3 pounds smoked ham hock or salt pork

Rinse beans, then pour them into a bowl or pot and cover with warm water. If you like, add two tablespoons of yogurt or whey and mix lightly. Cover and allow them to soak overnight. The next day, pour off the water, rinse beans thoroughly, and place them in a large, oven-proof pot or dutch oven (make sure it is coated cast iron). Pour in 2 quarts water, bring to a boil, and then simmer over low heat for one hour. Drain the beans once more. Return them to the large pot and add 1 quart water, plus all the remaining ingredients. Bring to a boil, then simmer, uncovered, over low heat for two hours. Preheat the oven to 300°. Cover the beans and roast them in the oven. When the beans are tender (usually after three hours), remove the lid and continue cooking them until the liquid is mostly evaporated and the beans are soft, generally an additional two hours.

If you are using salt pork, discard it before serving the beans. If you are using ham hocks, remove them, allow them to cool slightly, then pull off the skin to reveal the smoked meat. Pull off this meat and stir it into the beans before serving. Serves 6.

Note: Baked beans done in this style taste really wonderful when garnished with a small dollop of honey mustard.

Shannon Hayes
Warnerville, New York
shayes@midtel.net

SAP BUSH HOLLOW FARM'S
BRANDIED SHOULDER CHOPS WITH APRICOTS AND PRUNES

This is an easy crockpot recipe that kids and adults enjoy.

Herb Rub:
1 tablespoon dried sage
2 teaspoons dried thyme
1 tablespoon dried mustard
1 tablespoon salt
1 ½ teaspoons ground black pepper

4 pork shoulder chops or country-style ribs
1 onion, sliced into wedges
1 leek, finely sliced, white part only (optional)
3 to 4 carrots, chopped
½ cup pitted prunes
½ cup dried apricots
¼ cup sherry
1 cup beef or chicken stock
¼ cup brandy
2 bay leaves

Combine the herb rub ingredients and coat the chops. Cover with plastic wrap and refrigerate overnight, or let them sit 2 hours at room temperature. Place the onions, leeks, and carrots in the bottom of a large crockpot. Set the chops on top, then cover with the prunes and apricots. Pour in the sherry, stock, and brandy. Add bay leaves. Cook on low for 6 to 8 hours, until the meat falls away from the bones.

Shannon Hayes
Warnerville, New York
shayes@midtel.net

POULTRY & EGG RECIPES

GRAZEY ACRES'
CHICKEN WITH 40 CLOVES OF GARLIC

1 chicken (4 pounds, pastured broiler, of course)
6 tablespoons olive oil
salt and freshly ground pepper
3 sprigs fresh thyme
2 sprigs fresh rosemary
3 sprigs fresh sage
40 garlic cloves, unpeeled
12 whole black peppercorns
1 cup chicken broth
1 cup marsala wine

Preheat oven to 400 degrees. Rub outside of chicken with olive oil and season it inside and out with salt and pepper. Put half the thyme, rosemary and sage plus 10 garlic cloves in the cavity of the chicken. Place the chicken in a Dutch oven. Scatter remaining thyme, rosemary, sage, garlic, and peppercorns around the bird. Pour the broth in the bottom of the pan. Cover and bake for about 60 minutes, then remove the cover and let the bird brown for another 20 minutes. The total cooking time is about 20 minutes per pound of chicken.

Remove chicken from pan and place on a serving platter with garlic cloves. Put the pan with the drippings on the stovetop over high heat. Add the wine and scrape up any browned bits from the pan bottom, stirring constantly to reduce the sauce until it starts to thicken. Carve the meat and serve with a spoonful of sauce and a few cloves of garlic. *Note: The leftover carcass and drippings make an excellent broth.* Serves 4

Stacey and Jerry Muncie
Cory, Indiana
www.grazeyacres.com

SWEET GRASS FARM'S
HAPPY HEN STEW

1 large stewing chicken, approximately 4 ½ pounds
1 cup tomato juice
1 large onion, quartered
3 celery tops
3 celery ribs, cut into 1-inch pieces
1 bay leaf
5 carrots, sliced into coins
1 large tomato, diced
1 large green pepper, diced
1½ cups brown rice
1 cup small mushrooms
1 teaspoon curry powder
Pinch of dried tarragon

Cut chicken into serving pieces and simmer in a large kettle or Dutch oven with 2 cups of hot water, tomato juice, onion, celery tops, bay leaf, and 1 carrot. Simmer for 45 minutes.

Remove chicken pieces to a warm platter. Strain the broth, and skim off chicken fat. Return chicken pieces and broth to the kettle. Add all remaining ingredients, then add water or tomato juice to cover. Cook an additional hour, or until the rice is soft and chicken is tender. Serves 6.

Wendy Gornick
Vernon, New York
wgornick@born.com

DOMINION VALLEY FARM'S
LEMON HERB CHICKEN

¼ cup vegetable oil
¼ cup ketchup
2 tablespoons lemon juice
2 tablespoons soy sauce
¼ teaspoon salt
¼ teaspoon pepper
½ teaspoon rosemary leaves
½ teaspoon marjoram leaves
½ teaspoon thyme leaves
3 pounds chicken pieces, pasture-raised of course!
5 cups corn flakes or similar cereal, crushed to 3 cups

In a large mixing bowl, stir together oil, ketchup, lemon juice, soy sauce, salt, pepper, and herbs. Add chicken and turn to coat. Cover and refrigerate several hours, spooning marinade over chicken.

Drain chicken pieces slightly. Coat with cereal. Place in a single layer in shallow pan coated with vegetable cooking spray. Bake at 350 degrees for about an hour or until chicken is no longer pink. Do not cover pan or turn chicken while baking.

Brandon and Tammera Dykema
Allenton, Wisconsin
dominionvalleyfarm@juno.com
www.dominionvalleyfarm.com

SWEET GRASS FARM'S
SHERRIED CHICKEN LIVERS FOR PASTA

½ pound chicken livers, halved
2 tablespoons butter
½ cup dry sherry
¼ teaspoon rosemary
¼ teaspoon sage
¼ teaspoon black pepper
3 green onions, sliced

Sauté chicken livers in butter until they change color. Add dry sherry, rosemary, sage, black pepper, and green onions. Serve on cooked broad noodles tossed with oil. Serves 2 or 3.

Wendy Gornick

SWEET GRASS FARM'S
CHICKEN GIZZARD TREATS

These make great appetizers at informal backyard gatherings.

Chicken gizzards
Italian salad dressing

Marinate gizzards in Italian salad dressing for 30 minutes. Grill on moderately hot barbecue until done, taking care not to let them dry out.

Wendy Gornick
Vernon, New York
wgornick@born.com

FULL CIRCLE FARM'S
CHICKEN SALAD

This is our favorite chicken recipe. It is very flexible—add more or less of any one thing to your taste preference. We like it with lots of nuts and cream.

Meat from one pastured chicken, cut into pieces
1 cup mayonaise
½ to 1 cup cultured or regular cream, preferably raw from cows on
    green pasture
½ to 1 cup nuts (such as almonds, pecans or cashews), chopped
1 small apple, cored and cubed
1 stalk celery
½ medium onion, chopped
1 cup grapes cut in half or ½ cup raisins
1 tablespoon lemon juice
⅛ cup or more mustard
Salt, if desired

Mix all ingredients together. Serve on a piece of lettuce and add sliced tomato. Serves 6.

Dennis and Alicia Stoltzfoos
Dade City, Florida
thisisdennis@juno.com

DOMINION VALLEY FARM'S
DEER CAMP DUCK

One of our customers has an annual tradition of making a gourmet Thanksgiving dinner at deer camp with his hunting buddies. He was kind enough to share this recipe that we in turn have passed along to our customers. He says that the Dominion Valley Farm pasture-raised ducks were the best they have had in their years and years of deer camp!

8 to 10 pound Muscovy duck (or two smaller ducklings)
14–ounce bag seasoned bread stuffing
2 4–ounce cans mushroom pieces
1½ cups chopped onion
1½ cups chopped celery
⅛ cup finely chopped fresh garlic (about 8 to 10 cloves)
½ stick butter
2 to 3 bay leaves
Salt and pepper to taste

Discard liver and simmer neck and giblets in water with bay leaf for about 2 hours. Discard bay leaf and save liquid.

Cut up neck meat and giblets and mix into stuffing. Add butter to liquid and simmer until butter is melted. Mix in onion, celery, mushrooms, and garlic to stuffing. Add liquid gradually to stuffing until mixture is moist but not runny.

Season the duck inside and out with salt and pepper, then add stuffing mixture. Bake any excess stuffing wrapped in foil or in a baking dish during the last 1 hour of baking time.

Bake in covered pan with 1 cup of water on the bottom for approximately 2½ to 3 hours at 325 degrees. Uncover pan the last half-hour to brown the duck. The liquid in pan can be used to make gravy. Delicious served with cranberry sauce or cranberry chutney on the side.

Our five-month old son is too young to comment on these recipes, but they are favorites with our older boys ages three, four, and nine, who are all helpers in their own way in running our family business. We raise grassfed chickens, Muscovy ducks, turkey, Galloway beef, and Tamworth pigs.

Brandon and Tammera Dykema
Allenton, Wisconsin
dominionvalleyfarm@juno.com
www.dominionvalleyfarm.com

SAP BUSH HOLLOW FARM'S
DONEY'S EGGNOG

7 eggs
½ gallon milk
½ cup maple syrup
¼ teaspoon salt
2 tablespoons vanilla
2 cups whipped cream

Whisk together the eggs, milk, syrup, and salt in a large saucepan. Cook over low heat, stirring constantly, until the mixture thickens and coats a spoon, about one hour. Pour the mixture into a bowl and refrigerate for several hours.

The best way to enjoy wonderful grass-fed eggs and milk is in eggnog — not the junky stuff made with corn syrup that you find in the store, but real eggnog made with real eggs.

While this may traditionally be a holiday treat, my husband issues requests for it all year long. One taste of this stuff, and you'll understand why!
—Shannon Hayes

When you are ready to serve it, whip the cream and fold it into the eggnog. If you wish, stir in 1 cup rum and garnish with a few shakes of nutmeg.

Shannon Hayes
Warnerville, New York
shayes@midtel.net

SAUCES & RUBS RECIPES

KAMUELA PRIDE'S
JESSICA'S BRANDING FIRE RUB

This is a favorite on steak, grilled over the branding fire after our work is done, hence the name.

2 to 3 teaspoons chili powder

1 teaspoon paprika

1 teaspoon brown sugar

4 teaspoons Hawaiian or kosher salt

2 teaspoons cracked black pepper

1 to 2 teaspoons crushed red pepper

¼ teaspoon dry mustard

2 teaspoons dried garlic

1 teaspoon dried oregano leaves

"Branding time" is an old tradition still alive on many ranches, although not all of them continue the traditional branding process. The term encompasses all of the first work of the season's calves such as sorting, giving ear tags, etc.

Friends and neighbors lend a hand for the big work, and afterward join together around the fire for kaukau (food), music, and catching up since the last gathering. —Jan Dean

Combine all ingredients and mix thoroughly. Rub into meat and let sit at least five minutes – longer for stronger flavor – then grill, sear, or bake as desired. Store in airtight container. Rub will stay fresh longer if container is stored in the freezer.

Jan Dean, Kamuela Pride
Laupahoehoe, Hawaii
www.kamuelapride.com

NORDIC HILLS FARM'S
ZESTY BARBEQUE SAUCE FOR PASTURED MEATS

Serve sauce hot over spareribs, broiled chicken, short ribs, lamb chops, etc. I often parboil the ribs or chicken, then finish by basting liberally with the sauce and broiling or grilling them. Top the finished meat with more of the hot barbeque sauce.

¼ cup apple cider vinegar

½ cup water

2 tablespoons sugar

1 tablespoon prepared mustard

½ teaspoon freshly ground pepper

1½ teaspoons salt, preferably sea salt

¼ teaspoon cayenne pepper, or less if you prefer a milder sauce

1 thick slice of lemon or one tablespoon lemon juice

1 medium onion, sliced

¼ cup butter or olive oil

½ cup ketchup

2 tablespoons Worcestershire sauce

1½ teaspoons liquid smoke, optional

Mix vinegar, water, sugar, mustard, pepper, salt, cayenne, lemon, onion, and butter or olive oil together in a saucepan. Simmer uncovered for 20 minutes. Add ketchup, Worcestershire sauce and liquid smoke; bring to a boil.

We raise pastured poultry, lamb, beef and sometimes veal on our organic farm in southwestern Wisconsin's beautiful "coulee country." Our only crop is grass and our only reapers are our animals. We welcome visitors.

Jim and Mary Olsen
Ontario, Wisconsin
jim/maryolsen@centurytel.net

Notes and References
Recipe Index
General Index

Notes and References

Chapter 1   Imagine

1. Ward, G.M. P.L. Knox; B.W. Hobson. 1977. "Beef Production Options and Requirements for Fossil Fuel." Science 198(4314): 265-71.

Chapter 3   Down on the Pharm

1. "Broiler Chicken Skeletal Problems in the U.S."(A summary of information sources from 1990–2001.) United Poultry Concerns Fact Sheet

2. Papadopoulou, C., 1997, "Bacterial Strains Isolated from Eggs and Their Resistance to Currently Used Antibiotics: Is There a Health Hazard for Consumers?" Comp Immunol Microbiol Infect Dis 20, 1: 35-40.

Chapter 4   Exploring the Feed/Food Connection

1. Wolf, B. "Effects of Feeding a Return Chewing Gum/Packaging Material Mixture on Performance and Carcass Characteristics of Feedlot Cattle." 1996 J Anim Sci 74(11): 2559-65.

2. Rule, D. C., K. S. Broughton, S. M. Shellito, and G. Maiorano. 2002. "Comparison of Muscle Fatty Acid Profiles and Cholesterol Concentrations of Bison, Beef Cattle, Elk, and Chicken." J Anim Sci 80(5):1202-11.

No one study is the definitive reference for the difference in fat content between grass-fed and grain-fed cattle. There are a multitude of studies, each one using a slightly different protocol. But in general, the meat from grass-fed animals is much leaner than the meat from feedlot animals. In the study above, grain-fed animals had more than two and a half times more total fat in their meat than animals raised on grass.

3. Kang, J. X., and A. Leaf. (1996) "Antiarrhythmic Effects of Polyunsaturated Fatty Acids. Recent Studies." Circulation 94(7): 1774-80.

4. Hu, F. B., M. J. Stampfer, *et al.* (1999). "Dietary intake of alpha-linolenic acid and risk of fatal ischemic heart disease among women." <u>Am J Clin Nutr</u> 69(5): 890-7.

5. T. A. Dolecek and G. Granditis, (1991) "Dietary Polyunsaturated FattyAcids and Mortality in the Multiple Risk Factor Inter-ventionTrial (Mrfit)," <u>World Rev Nutr Diet</u> 66:205-16.

6. The *www.eatwild.com* website has a comprehensive list of studies comparing the amount of omega-3s in grass-fed with the amount in grain-fed animals. Look for the "Scientific Research" section.

✓ 7. Simopoulos, A. P. 'The Importance of the Ratio of Omega-6/ Omega-3 Essential Fatty Acids." (2002). <u>Biomed Pharmacother</u> 56 (8): 365-79.

   Also, read The Omega Diet, *the book I co-authored with Simopoulos. It features an in-depth exploration of EFAs.*

✓ 8. Eaton, S. B., and S. B. Eaton, 3rd. (2000). "Paleolithic Vs. Modern Diets—Selected Pathophysiological Implications" <u>Eur J Nutr</u> 39, (2):67-70.

9. Visit the Scientific References section of www.eatwild.com for a studies on EFA ratios in meat, eggs, and dairy products.

10. Dhiman, T. R., G. R. Anand, L. D. Satter, and M. W. Pariza. (1999). "Conjugated Linoleic Acid Content of Milk from Cows Fed Different Diets." <u>J Dairy Sci</u> 82, (10): 2146-56.

   French, P., C. Stanton, F. Lawless, E. G. O'Riordan, F. J. Monahan, P. J. Caffrey, and A. P. Moloney. (2003) "Fatty Acid Composition, Including Conjugated Linoleic Acid, of Intramuscu-lar Fat from Steers Offered Grazed Grass, Grass Silage, or Concentrate-Based Diets." <u>J Anim Sci</u> 78, (11): 2849-55.

   Visit the Scientific References section of *www.eatwild.com* for additional CLA studies.

11. Lavillonniere, F., and P. Bougnoux. (2003) "Dietary Purified Cis-9,Trans-11 Conjugated Linoleic Acid Isomer Has Anticarcino-genic Properties in Chemically Induced Mammary Tumors in Rats." <u>Nutr Cancer</u> 45(2):190-4.

Many studies have looked at the effect of CLA on cancer in animals. Only recently have studies focused on the isomer of CLA found in animals. Studies such as this one give a better indication of the possible effects of eating grass-fed products rich in CLA.

12. Stanton, Catherine *et al.* Armis No. 4257. The Dairy Products Research Centre, Moorepark, Ireland. ISBN 1-84170 118 1

13. Aro, A., S. Mannisto, I. Salminen, M. L. Ovaskainen, V. Kataja, and M. Uusitupa. (2002) "Inverse Association between Dietary and Serum Conjugated Linoleic Acid and Risk of Breast Cancer in Postmenopausal Women." Nutr Cancer 38: 151-7.

14. Kritchevsky, D., S. A. Tepper, S. Wright, P. Tso, and S. K. Czarnecki. (2000). "Influence of Conjugated Linoleic Acid (CLA) on Establishment and Progression of Atherosclerosis in Rabbits." J Am Coll Nutr 19: 472S-77S.

15. Noone, E. J., H. M. Roche, A. P. Nugent, and M. J. Gibney. (2002) "The Effect of Dietary Supplementation Using Isomeric Blends of Conjugated Linoleic Acid on Lipid Metabolism in Healthy Human Subjects." Br J Nutr 88 (3): 243-51.

It's important to note that the CLA that produced these results was a 80/20 blend of the type of CLA found in grazing animals and a type that occurs in very small amounts, "trans-10,cis-12 CLA."

16. Tolan, A., J. Robertson, C. R. Orton, M. J. Head, A. A. Christie, and B. A. Millburn. (1974) "Studies on the Composition of Food. The Chemical Composition of Eggs Produced under Battery, Deep Litter and Free Range Conditions." Br J Nutr 31 (2):185-200.

17. Simopoulos, A. P. and N. Salem, Jr. (1989). "n-3 fatty acids in eggs from range-fed Greek chickens." N Engl J Med 321(20): 1412.

Chapter 5   Grass-Fed Beef: One of the Healthiest Foods on the Menu

1. Hermel, S.R. (1993). "Extending the bloom. By extending the cherry-red color of beef, vitamin E could help boost sales all

around." *Beef Magazine.* 8-12.

2. Smith, G.C. "Dietary Supplementation of Vitamin E to Cattle to Improve Shelf-Life and Case-Life for Domestic and International Markets." Colorado State University. Complete reference not known.

3. Prache, S., A. Priolo, *et al.* (2003). "Persistence of carotenoid pigments in the blood of concentrate-finished grazing sheep: its significance for the traceability of grass-feeding." J Anim Sci 81(2): 360-7.

4. Nader, Glenn and Steve Blank. "Thinking through the process: grass-fed beef." University of California Sustainable Agriculture Research and Education Program.

5. Toniolo, P., A. L. Van Kappel, *et al.* (2001). "Serum carotenoids and breast cancer." Am J Epidemiol 153(12): 1142-7.

6. Rule, D. C., K. S. Broughton, S. M. Shellito, and G. Maiorano. (2002) "Comparison of Muscle Fatty Acid Profiles and Cholesterol Concentrations of Bison, Beef Cattle, Elk, and Chicken." J Anim Sci 80(5):1202-11.

Chapter 6   Super Healthy Milk

1. Dhiman, T. R., G. R. Anand, L. D. Satter, and M. W. Pariza. (1999) "Conjugated Linoleic Acid Content of Milk from Cows Fed Different Diets." J Dairy Sci 82 (10): 2146-56.

2. Searles, S. K., and J. G. Armstrong. (1970) "Vitamin E, Vitamin A, and Carotene Contents of Alberta Butter." *J Dairy Sci* 53 (2): 150-4.

3. Jensen, S. K., A. K. Johannsen, and J. E. Hermansen. (1999) "Quantitative Secretion and Maximal Secretion Capacity of Retinol,Beta-Carotene and Alpha-Tocopherol into Cows' Milk." J Dairy Res 66(4): 511-22.

Chapter 7   Grass-Fed Bison, Lamb, and Pork

1. Rule, D. C., K. S. Broughton, *et al.* (2002). "Comparison of muscle fatty acid profiles and cholesterol concentrations of bison, beef cattle, elk, and chicken." J Anim Sci 80(5): 1202-11.

2. Wolf, B. W., E. C. Titgemeyer, L. L. Berger, and G. C. Fahey, Jr. (1994) "Effects of Chemically Treated, Recycled Newsprint on Feed Intake and Nutrient Digestibility by Growing Lambs." J Anim Sci 72(9): 2508-17.

   Cooke, J. A., and J. P. Fontenot. (1990) "Utilization of Phosphorus and Certain Other Minerals from Swine Waste and Broiler Litter." J Anim Sci 68(9):2852-63.

3. Pearce, J., and D. M. Chestnutt. (1974) "A Comparison of the Fatty Acid Composition of Adipose Tissue Triglyceride from Grass-Fed and Intensively-Reared Lambs." Proc Nutr Soc 33 (3): 99A-100A.

4. Prache, S., A. Priolo, et al. (2003). "Persistence of carotenoid pigments in the blood of concentrate-finished grazing sheep: its significance for the traceability of grass-feeding." J Anim Sci 81(2): 360-7.

5. Ray, E. E., R. P. Kromann, et al. (1975). "Relationships between fatty acid composition of lamb fat and dietary ingredients." J Anim Sci 41(6): 1767-74

6. "The Multiple Benefits of Agriculture – An Economic, Environmental and Social Analysis, November 2001." Produced by the Land Stewardship Project, White Bear Lake, Minnesota.

7. "Livestock Confinement Dust And Gases" produced by Iowa State University Extension and published in the National Agriculture Safety Database. Available on the Internet at http://www.cdc.gov/nasd/docs/d001501-d001600/d001501/d001501.html

8. Koizumi, I., Y. Suzuki, and J. J. Kaneko. (1991) "Studies on the Fatty Acid Composition of Intramuscular Lipids of Cattle, Pigs and Birds." J Nutr Sci Vitaminol (Tokyo) 37(6):545-54.

Chapter 8   Free-Living Poultry

1. Simopoulos, A. P. and N. Salem, Jr. (1989). "n-3 fatty acids in eggs from range-fed Greek chickens." N Engl J Med 321(20): 1412.

2. Barbara Gorski obtained a SARE grant to analyze eggs and chickens from her Double G Farm and two neighboring, Forks Farm and the Lone Pine Farm.

Chapter 9   Where Do You Find It? How Do You Cook It?

1. Hardin, Ben. "Predicting Tenderness in Beefsteaks" Agricultural Research, November 1999. [Note: Agricultural Research is a USDA publication.]

Recipe Index

Index